LIVING WITH MANIA

By Dick Redbourn

"One million people commit suicide every year."

The World Health Organization

Published by:
Chipmunkapublishing
PO Box 6872
Brentwood
Essex
CM13 1ZT
United Kingdom

www.chipmunkapublishing.com

FOREWORD

A detailed personal account of 25 years living with mania, the 'high side' form of manic depression. It includes the main events in my mental history, details of the periods during and around my two formal breakdowns, and my efforts to cope with the many manic episodes. More recently, I report on my reduced ability to cope with continuous concentration and/or fast data inflow to the brain.

In five appendices, I analyse the component structure of the manic episode; my lifestyle ideas for coping; the social problem; a comparison with the formal definition of mania; and final reflections.

INTRODUCTION

My life as a grammar school boy in the '50s was dominated by sport; it seemed playing games was of at least comparable importance to study. Nevertheless, we were much encouraged to strive for a university place, supposedly the key to a future life of affluence. In unspectacular fashion I achieved this, and by the time we'd moved into the '60s — coinciding with my twenties — I'd settled for physics at college and cricket as my sporting passion.

The '60s are famously recalled as the decade of sex, drugs and rock 'n' roll, most of which seemed to pass me by, or happen in another place. It was still necessary for 'ordinary' people to earn their living, mostly in an unexciting and conventional way.

Having graduated from Durham University with a degree in pure physics, I drifted into what is now known as Building Services engineering. I decided to train and specialise in air conditioning, believing — wrongly! — it had a great future in this country.

After working for contractors and consultants for a few years, since '67 I've been involved with equipment manufacturers. If I'm expert in anything, it's in a very narrow engineering field: the design, costing and competitive tendering of customised air handling and packaged air conditioning equipment. Enough said!

Cricket suited me perfectly; the ritual, characters, trips to the country grounds, and after-match sessions in the pub dominated my summer weekends. It is also the ideal game for an observer - someone who likes to savour the whole scene, with its funny incidents and anecdotes, then squirrel them away to memory. With much practice, I've now learnt to develop and exaggerate a minor detail into a full-blown humorous story, to be frequently re-told at great length!

My fun from cricket reached its peak in the early '70s and, anxious not to forget the lovely stories, I decided to write a book. I scribbled them down over a year, then punted the finished article around for another year to find a publisher. Eventually 'The Domestic Cricketer' was launched with due fanfare in '77, and didn't quite sink without trace.

I continued playing 'the greatest game' until August '92, when I reluctantly decided to hang up my boots. For me It was a particularly sad and rather frightening occasion, active sport having played such a prominent part of my life. In fact, I'd long believed the day I stopped playing 'running-about games' would mark the end of my worthwhile existence.

Initially in my 'after-life' I wasn't sure what to do next; golf then bowls is the usual route. There were reasons why I didn't want to go down that road so, by '94 and anxious to get on with something, I decided to revisit my book. I'd always thought I could've made a better job if I'd taken more time so, with much extra material available, I decided to construct a full-length, humorous autobiography.

It took over two years to write and gave me tremendous pleasure as I wrestled to knit all the anecdotes, stories and characters together. 'Cricket at the Grassroots', self-published in April '96 without advertising, sold 'modestly', but I recovered most of my financial outlay.

At that point, with my 'problem', I came to the conclusion that writing was an ideal hobby for me. Uninterested in fiction (and certainly unable to write any), I've long been fascinated by journalism, with its need to convey information quickly and concisely.

I'd never suggest I'm a writer, just an amateur scribbler, and would loathe to get involved in the unpleasant business of having to hit deadlines. But for me, writing has therapeutic value, allowing me to exercise my mind at the pace I choose, and I much enjoy selecting the most apposite words in piecing together the final text, like a giant jigsaw puzzle.

Having exhausted cricket, by '97 I was looking for something else to write about. Apart from my professional knowledge as an engineer, the only subject possible was my twenty plus years living with mania.

After rudimentary research, I decided to tackle this topic, aware that there couldn't be a much bigger contrast for a scribbler than moving from sporting humour to mental illness. With such a complex subject, I started in '98 by making notes about my mental history and have kept a diary of all relevant events since then.

Initial searches of the internet showed that mania falls within the category of mental illness, long known to the general public as 'manic depression'. It was renamed some years ago as 'bipolar affective disorder', but now seems to be called 'bipolar disorder'. As for how many suffer from this illness, I found a whole spread of figures, but the one most frequently quoted is 'one percent of the population'. *1

As most people are aware, people with this illness have mood swings which alternate between the 'high' side (mania) and the 'low' side (depression). There appear to be many variations on the basic disorder with Bipolar 1, Bipolar 2, Mixed states, etc. I can't be too certain under which category I should be classified, but would reckon 'unipolar manic, or hypomanic' to be a fair description. *2

There is a British and European protocol on mental health (ICD10), whose standards and definitions run parallel with those of the American Psychiatric Association (APA), originators of the 'Diagnostic and Statistical Manual of Mental Disorders' (DSM). For my convenience, as more comprehensive information is available, I've used the American DSM standard when making comparisons in this paper (as in Appendix D).

In the 4th Edition (DSM-IV, 1994) the APA omitted the category of people who suffer from mania only, presumably relegating the problem below the official list of disorders.

I found an interesting quote about this from an expert commentator:

*'There are a few rare documented cases of mania without depression, but DSM-IV does not currently include a category for just "mania". (This diagnosis was present in DSM-III, but is unaccountably absent in DSM-IV!) *3*

This seems to have been a somewhat controversial revision, and one much discussed and debated by the experts. Whatever the technicalities, it's given me an added incentive to record my experiences, and goes some way to explain why I've never met, or even heard about, anyone else with exactly the same problem as myself.

Another reason to put on record my manic experiences, and efforts to cope with them, is simply that I've put hundreds, probably thousands, of hours of thought into the subject. Without delusions of grandeur (!), it's just possible one or two of my ideas might be of interest to others.

I've read one or two autobiographical books on bipolar disorder, to give myself an idea of the way the subject has been tackled. Particularly noticeable were regular passages of high-blown rhetoric and dramatic, emotional trauma. Although possibly an accurate recollection of events, there seemed little attempt at detailed self-analysis, or consideration of lifestyle changes. I got the impression that the authors believed these things best left to medication and psychiatric advice - and of course that may well have been right.

I assume my character and personality must have played some part in my mental troubles. Clearly I am an introverted person, constantly analysing and correcting my actions through my years with mania, though this might be considered a positive advantage.

Going through university at a time when only two percent of the population did so gave me an underlying core of self-confidence which has never diminished. It also instilled a lifelong interest in science and belief in the scientific method - without meaning to imply that this account belongs in that category!

Verbally I've developed a style encompassing self-deprecation, defeatism, an almost feudal reactionism*4, and sentimentality. As well as establishing personality, it's of great value for generating humour - a sure-fire way to relax people and defuse tension.

This leads on to my 'theory' about non-clinical depression; it must surely have some connection with optimism and pessimism. For as long as I can remember I've been a pessimist, growing more cynical over the years, a state of mind viewed as sad (even pathetic) by many 'get up and go' optimists. Yet logically it must be a sensible and practical approach to life - If you expect the worst to happen, whatever transpires must be better! Disappointment, with the possibility of depression, is minimised, and one moves through life without a trail of shattered hopes. (Taking chances is another matter; I realise there's no excitement or gain without risk.)

Furthermore, if my spirits droop and I do become slightly depressed, I rationalise objectively to put my situation into perspective. At the outer level, I live in one of the most civilised, peaceful, affluent and democratic parts of the world. At the personal level, I have a home, a loving family, good physical health, a job and many friends to protect me from the rigours outside, as well as fulfilling all my material and emotional needs.

I'm aware that the above statements might be dicing with fate, and some disaster may befall me tomorrow, wiping out much that I cherish. But the future cannot change the past; with three score years under my belt I can now look back with great pleasure at all the fun and good fortune I've had.

My broad objective in this account is to write down everything that may be relevant to my problems with mania, explain my reasoning, and detail my actions to reduce the effects of those problems. To lighten things up (if possible!), I'll include any amusing anecdotes along the way.

I have no medical or psychiatric training, or any qualification to help me in tackling this task. I shall use some fairly obvious pseudo-technical terms, such as: adrenaline up, going high, head temperature, over the top, delusions, cooled down, washed out, etc. The key term I will use refers to the cycle from normality into mania and back, which I believe is correctly called a 'manic episode'.

Finally, I've not named the many medical professionals who've grappled with me over the years. My opinion of their performance, particularly during my more manic periods, must be considered 'somewhat unreliable'!

Childhood

I understand there's a school of thought among psychiatrists that tensions and stress endured by a pregnant woman can be transmitted to the child in the womb. True or false, my mother could not have carried me through a much more traumatic time - the darkest days of the Second World War in 1940.

I was born at home in Brighton (under the bombers' route to London) in the early morning of one of the first day-night raids of the Battle of Britain — I've always felt a quite irrational tinge of pride about that. I've few memories of the war of course and, although the odd bomb fell nearby, got through it without harm.

In '46 I started at Balfour Road School and went through my primary education with just one strong memory: my mother rushing to buy mangy outer leaves of cabbage from the local greengrocer, as she struggled to feed the five of us. School food was awful and my mother tried to provide all my meals from home, but during the period of official food rationing, that was easier said than done. The legacy of all that is that even now I have great difficulty in leaving food on the plate.

I took and passed the 11 plus exam in '51 and moved on to Varndean Grammar School for Boys for my secondary education. With a combination of sport and (some!) study I went through eight happy years to the sixth form, finishing as Senior Prefect, before gaining a place at Durham University in '59.

I can't remember doing anything in my childhood to suggest future mental problems: I was brought up with three sisters, in a secure and loving home, by parents reasonably happily married and much devoted to their children.

None of my close family have had any history of mental troubles, and when I traced my ancestors back to the mid-nineteenth century, I found nothing in either line to suggest there might be. There's no obvious link therefore to the possibility of inherited genes, or any evidence of mania.

The Durham Event

In my second year at Durham University I was involved in a traumatic event, the essential details of which I can recall quite clearly even now. It's the one part of this account which can make me feel quite emotional.

I returned home for the Christmas break in December '60, a few days before a serious outbreak of smallpox, centred on Bradford, was announced. My mother had always been strongly against vaccinations, or jabs of any sort, so I'd had none since the day I was born. But at that time there was no option; the College authorities stated that no students would be allowed to return without a vaccination.

I had the jab a few days before returning to Durham, then a week later (stupidly perhaps) I played in a tough soccer match after which I went to bed feeling feverish.

Overnight I became sweaty and light headed, and with no medical facilities in the College, my Tutor decided to send me to Dryburn County Hospital for observation.

I was put into a men's general ward, populated mostly by miners suffering from advanced respiratory diseases. In the bed next to me was a man who had to be restrained in a cot as he rolled around in the terminal stage of Bright's disease, an image I will never forget. He had a coughing fit every minute or so, without respite, and died on my fourth day there.

The noise in the ward was continual: coughing, wailing and staff coming and going. The lights were kept on constantly, with a large red one right over my bed. For a 'soft southerner' who'd never been in hospital before, it was all, quite literally, a nightmare.

To my intense frustration, everything conspired against all that I really needed - peace and quiet, so I could get a decent night's sleep. I knew I was being given strong sedatives, yet recall wandering about the ward in the early hours, wide awake, praying I would start to feel drowsy.

It was usually around 5 in the morning before I finally collapsed into an exhausted sleep. Then came the cruel part: at 6 o'clock sharp, a chap wheeling a noisy, industrial cleaner started his round. If the noise alone didn't wake me, he'd jerk each bed roughly to one side to reach the floor underneath. Soon after, the morning routine of washing, breakfast, pills, bed-making and so on would unfold, making even a light doze impossible.

My parents had not been contacted as I'd begged the hospital staff not to do so, fearing the news might cause them unnecessary alarm. So no one from outside was aware of my situation, with its steady decline from sleep deprivation into delusions and delirium.

After a week, the Dryburn authorities decided they couldn't handle me and I was transferred to Chester-le-Street Psychiatric Hospital. *5

Again I was put into a large, male ward, this time with inmates permanently deranged, mostly middle-aged or older. Many had been there for years and simply wandered about the place day and night, muttering to themselves, punctuated with the odd shout.   In crude jargon, I was in the 'loony bin' or 'cuckoo's nest'.

A heavy course of sodium amytal was prescribed for me, which I found most unnerving.   I lost any calculated subtlety, tact or inhibitions; I simply thought, spoke and behaved exactly as I felt.   One morning I woke up startled, convinced I was Jesus Christ arriving for the second coming! Whatever else, this induced a glowing sense of triumph, warmth and relief, and relaxed me enough to allow some sleep.

In the state I was in, it was only to be expected that people looked at me in amazement, if not wonder. With hindsight, it was my first experience of the disconcerting 'staring effect', with which I became well acquainted during manic episodes years later.

An amusing incident at this time, illustrating my state of mind, occurred when three of my College pals decided to visit me one evening. Students rarely had cars in those days, so the journey from Durham was quite a trek.   They walked to the bus station, rode for seven miles and then trudged another half mile through snow and ice.

When they finally arrived, my pals burst into the room for the hour's visiting time, full of sparkle, bounce and wit, determined to brighten my day.   I was lying in bed, half buried under the sheets, feeling totally washed out when I was hit with this gale of high spirits.   I tried to respond in kind but after less than two minutes felt utterly exhausted, just wanting peace and quiet.

I cringed and shut my eyes till they stopped talking, when they realised something was wrong.   As they peered at me with concern I could only whisper, reflecting my true feelings, 'will you go away please!'. Two understood, but my third pal was most upset, almost ready to start an argument; 'Cor crikey, I've come all this bloody way just for two minutes!' He had to be ushered out, dragged almost, still protesting about the waste of time.

After three days at Chester-le-Street, I reluctantly agreed that my parents be told about my problems, and a letter was sent immediately. On receiving the news they were naturally most shocked and alarmed; but my father simply put his hat and coat on, grabbed some pillows and blankets and drove to Durham. (That was quite an ordeal before motorways; 310 miles in snow and ice, in a car manufactured in the '40s).

When he came into the ward I was immensely relieved, to say the least, while he was equally stunned to hear the gibberish I was spouting. For some hours he couldn't understand what was going on as the medical staff explained that I was seriously, mentally ill. The best hope of a cure, they told him, was an intensive six-week course of drugs, to start immediately.

Having left school at 13 with minimal education, and in an age of almost unqualified deference to the medical profession, it took great courage on my father's part to say 'no' to this proposal and insist I be discharged immediately. But he did just that, bundled me into the back of the car and drove back to Brighton as quickly as possible.

Within minutes of returning home I was in bed and slept for nearly 24 hours. After three days of rest and sleep I felt more or less back to normal and keen to return to College.

Of course it wasn't that simple; officialdom was involved. The College authorities stated I couldn't return that academic year due to the proximity of Finals, and so would have to wait till October to re-start my final year.

Irrational though it may be, nothing will ever dissuade me that my father's prompt and decisive actions not only enabled me to make a full recovery, but saved me from becoming a long-term — lifelong, even — inmate in a mental institution. I'm pleased I remembered to thank him again, shortly before he sank into Alzheimer's, a few months before his death.

There is a humorous postscript to this affair. Before I was allowed to go back to College for the next year, I had to be given the 'all-clear' by a supposedly top Harley Street psychiatrist.

It was actually most important that I got through this test, as to lose another year may have meant I lost interest altogether. So, on the appointed day, I donned my best suit and travelled to London, in good time for the appointment. Reaching Harley Street I recall being amazed by the number of Rolls and Bentleys parked or double-parked in the road, as I strode along, peering at the gleaming brass plate beside each front door.

Having found the place and been ushered in by an all-white clad nurse, I sat in the waiting room, in cathedral-like silence. I was eventually shown into a large consulting room, complete with antique desk, bookshelves and so on, but dominated by an imposing, long, leather couch. This was a touch intimidating and I imagined I'd soon be stretched out full length, as the psychiatrist deftly probed the innermost recesses of my mind.

In fact the psychiatrist, probably in his mid-thirties, spent a great deal of time fussily measuring my height and weight using some ancient, dilapidated equipment. He couldn't get the level pointer to stay put before he took a height reading and became increasingly frustrated about this. Then he asked for a 'sample' and I had to perform, behind a screen, into a large, white, enamelled wash bowl.

I reckoned afterwards all this took nearly half the interview time, before he moved on to a few gentle, general questions. Then the big moment; he announced he intended to do a Rorschach (inkblot) test. He explained he'd show me 10 cards, in sequence, each with a splattered inky image on it and I had to tell him the first thing that came to mind.

I got myself all psyched up, but the first one was simple, 'a beetle'. I thought the second looked similar so I said, 'a spider'. Then I opted for a 'crushed beetle', a 'dead fly' and so on till only on the ninth did I manage a dramatic switch to 'railway cuttings'. Immediately I spoilt this by following up with 'an aerial view of railway cuttings'. In all I'd identified eight insects in various stages of disfigurement and two railway cuttings. I knew I'd performed badly.

He then took out a sort of 'crib sheet' and proceeded to go into lengthy calculations. When he got to the end of these he sat there shaking his head, as if to indicate he must've got something wrong. So he went through it all again and once more shook his head in disbelief.

I was becoming alarmed; it seemed I was either the greatest genius since Einstein or a raving idiot, but nothing in between. He then checked the sums yet again, finally confident he was right. For some moments he sat struggling to find the right words to phrase his verdict as tactfully as possible. I sat goggle-eyed in anticipation until at last he pronounced: 'I'm sorry, but I'm afraid it looks as if you've got virtually no imagination whatsoever!'

Although deflated, I wasn't too hurt or worried about this at the time; I saw no reason why this should prevent my return to College. But I pondered more deeply about what it all meant on the train back to Brighton. Clearly, becoming a novelist or surrealist painter was out, but I didn't see why it should stop me playing cricket and football! But seriously, it did have a deeper psychological effect: during the forty years since, I've always assumed I've got no imagination, and never bothered to try anything that would appear to need any. It's remained my 'received wisdom', for the simple reason that I've neither sought nor received any other opinion on the matter.

When everything died down after the Durham episode, the medical authorities were slow to issue their report on what precisely had happened. My father was anxious that I avoid any stigma associated with a mental breakdown, particularly at that stage of my career. Various 'discussions' took place, the details of which I had no knowledge; when the final report emerged, it stated that I'd had 'severe vaccine fever'.

This slightly furtive debate sowed some doubt in my mind for some years after as to what had really happened. But much later on, having actually experienced breakdowns, it became obvious that exhaustion due to sleep deprivation had caused delusions. The very fact I'd recovered so rapidly made it certain I hadn't suffered a breakdown.

When all the above was put behind me, I returned for my last year and took my finals as planned. Like most students, I left revision to the last moment and worked at a frenzied pace during the summer months to make up time.

I clearly remember my last three-hour exam paper, which I struggled to finish. My friends gathered outside afterwards in high spirits; a visit to the local pub was readily and enthusiastically agreed. But I felt exhausted and my head was hot so I went back to my room to rest. I was too 'hot' to doze or sleep but to get peace I just read for several hours.

Although I thought nothing of it at the time, it was the first occasion I can recall when something arose to suggest that I might lack mental strength or stamina; or to put it another way, was there a problem waiting to happen?

Young adult

The 16 years from leaving University up to my first formal breakdown in '79 passed without any obvious mental problems. There were no repercussions from the Durham event and I did all the things one does at that stage of life: got on with my career, got married and started a family. *6

I'd decided to go into air conditioning engineering for my career, and so attended night school in London for technical training. There was one part of my studies, of relevance to this account, which I've always remembered. The principle aim of an air conditioning system is, of course, to produce the optimum temperature and humidity levels in the occupied space, called the 'comfort zone'. There are a host of additional factors that influence this; individual characteristics, activity level, clothing, air movement, etc. But apart from this, the basic physiology of the human being dictates that, with high blood flow and biochemical activity, the head generates — and has to dispose of — more heat than any other part of the body. This leads to an optimum balancing air temperature surrounding the head of about 16C. Conversely, the feet and hands, with relatively low blood flow and large surface area, are in balance around 27C.

It's possible to get somewhere near these conditions for most periods of the year in our temperate climate. When outside, with head uncovered and judicious use of clothing for the extremities, one can achieve the right sort of temperature difference. Likewise, indoors in winter, by turning the design temperature setting down and using more clothing, a reasonable comfort level can be obtained.

Later on, when I started my struggles with mania, I became acutely aware of this temperature balance and have always made great efforts since to keep my head cool. This has conferred the additional benefit of providing welcome temporary relief from the distressing 'hot head' feeling, when over-tense. *7

Soon after I left Durham I joined St James's, an old-established cricket club playing in the Brighton area. In truth I wasn't a particularly good player, having had no proper coaching at school, but I soon became hooked on the club cricket scene, St James's in particular, and was keen to make an impression with my new colleagues.

After a match we'd congregate in a pub for a drinks session for a couple of hours. Any contentious points in the game were debated and old stories were re-told, with jokes and much repartee. This part of the ritual I especially enjoyed; I was anxious to make my mark somehow, and as I wasn't contributing much on the field of play, I quickly learnt to think and talk fast on my feet.

As the years passed it became something I could switch on at will, and I kept this Groucho Marx style of talking for use at parties or any social event, to help generate a more exciting, boisterous atmosphere. At the same time, an accelerated thought process had crept into my job as, for the first time, I came under increasing pressure at work.

I'm sure the '70s were the incubation period for my first breakdown, and I shall describe what I think were the contributory factors. But first, the word 'stress': the word is much bandied about and over-used today, and as such I would never claim to be under any greater pressure than the rest of the working population. But then, of course, all things are relative, and some people are better equipped to deal with a particular level or type of stress than others.

I've been lucky with my home life; I married Carol in '68 and our two children, Lisa and Mark, were born in '69 and '71. There were no problems with their health and early years and I've enjoyed a happy marriage to date. (In my domestic life therefore, there's been no obvious change in my basic stress level.)

In the deeper sense however, there was one underlying tension I was obliged to shoulder, again like millions of others. As the only family breadwinner, I was acutely aware of my responsibility to 'bring home the bacon'. I'd have been appalled to let my children down, or cause a substantial reduction in their living standard, by failing in this prime task.

By the mid-'70s I had become well established as a designer and estimator in a small firm of air conditioning equipment manufacturers in Crowborough. We were expanding rapidly, leading to staff becoming over-stretched; often I had to do secretarial jobs, answer the phone, copying, sending letters and so on, on top of my basic job. The offices were usually undersized, with ancient desks, limited shelving and no filing systems - oh, and of course, with no proper ventilation or air conditioning!

The absence of a decent filing system may seem trivial but it meant I'd try to keep pertinent facts about jobs in my head. Though this was quicker for me, it also meant colleagues found it simpler to ask me than delve into an untidy job file. There were regular interruptions from works staff - querying drawings, asking for more details, or requesting my presence to look at a problem on the shop floor - and as the office was part of the factory area, the noise generated by drilling, hammering and moving large metal equipment was a regular source of irritation.

In that environment I had to try and concentrate on my main function: the equipment design, costing and preparation of quotations for clients. The overriding problem all estimators faced then, and even more so now, is that of the deadline. Interruptions, delays in obtaining information, panics on other projects and staff problems effectively increase the work load with no increase in the time available to complete the job.

The obvious physical analogy for this is that of a juggler, trying to keep a dozen balls in the air at once, with increasing speed, while people around are doing their best to distract him. When a big project was finished I'd feel I'd been 'through the ringer' mentally, and be tired for some days; at the time however, I never gave any thought to the possibility of this process causing long-term health problems. With hindsight I'm quite certain that this practice, repeated regularly, set up my breakdown and subsequent struggles with mania.

In my early days as a sportsman, I'd taken great delight in discovering the limits of my physical strength and stamina. Yet in spite of that experience, at no time till after my first breakdown did I even consider there might be equivalent limits of my mental abilities. This obvious oversight meant I paid no notice to a number of incidents that may have been minor (submerged?) manic episodes.

On one occasion I became hysterical with laughter over something no one else found funny, then fainted for several seconds. When my first cricket book was finished the effort left me exhausted and several times I became tearful and went into a limp, shocked state. When I later experienced this condition on another occasion I instinctively did the right thing: rested and kept quiet until my mental strength was restored. All these things were of a minor, fleeting nature, and appeared to have had no lasting effects.

The only behaviour that caused comment was my extremely placid nature and refusal to get involved in a 'shouting match', whatever the provocation. When I discussed this with my GP, he said it was better to relieve stress by anger. In a confrontation, therefore, I should fight back to raise the tension, thereby burning off adrenaline.

(Somehow, I was never happy with that advice. I've always avoided arguments, rationalising that if the other person's wrong, it doesn't matter much. If they're right, it's best to recognise the situation and sort it out with an apology.

I believe this has been a subject of long-running debate in the psychiatric world, only recently resolved in favour of the non-confrontational approach. Apart from what's best for 'normal' people, in my case I've instinctively felt arguments — leading to 'rage' perhaps — must heighten my adrenaline level and bring forward the onset of another manic episode. It therefore appears that I've always practised what's now accepted as the best option.)

Not long before my first breakdown there were two abnormal events which may have been of significance in adding to my stress level. In September '79 my mother-in-law died of cancer, having been nursed at home through the final weeks by her daughters. Contrary to stereotype, I had great respect and affection for her, and although I was shielded from the anguish of the last days, the trauma of it all was distressing.

Secondly, for some years I'd been the technical director of the air conditioning manufacturers in Crowborough where I worked. During the good times we'd built up staff to around 80, but then a calamitous work shortage meant half the employees had to be made redundant after the Christmas break of '78. Although not directly responsible, I felt I should shoulder part of the blame, which left me nursing a sense of guilt for some time.

Notwithstanding all this, I can't say that I had any idea, or noticed anything unusual, to suggest that I was heading for a mental breakdown. Apart from the last few weeks, I remained blissfully unaware of all the stresses and tensions that must have been building up in my mind. Even today, with much greater experience of these things, I doubt I'd have been able to anticipate or avoid this traumatic event.

The first breakdown

The rapid build-up to my first breakdown was during January '79, a period of which I remember little. Carol had noticed my behaviour becoming stranger by the day; I seemed troubled and much preoccupied with my own thoughts. Difficulty with sleeping led to a visit to my GP, who prescribed sleeping pills and tranquillisers, to little effect.

In the week before my admission to hospital, I was waking in the early morning, in tears, with an intense head pain. The best, in fact the only, description of this I can offer, is that it felt like an iron band clamped tightly round my forehead. I would clutch hands to my head to try and relieve the tension and initially, I thought it might be a physical problem. Certainly we were both bewildered as to what was happening.

With experience, I've since learnt to recognise the features of a manic episode, and I now believe I was in the middle of a major one at that time. One symptom I can still remember - a powerful one - I now call the 'staring effect', and I shall describe it in detail later. At the time of my breakdown I believed everyone on television was addressing their remarks to me personally; even the news bulletins had been tailor-made for my viewing! This delusion lasted for some time and was the cause of great concern to Carol and our friends.

As I moved to the climax of the manic episode (or episodes?), the delusions became stronger, and totally took over my mind. I've since found that there's usually one substantive theme in each episode. But during this breakdown there seemed to be at least three concurrent delusions, each driving me 'over the top'.

Firstly, I developed a 'theory' about black holes and the end of the universe. Then I wrote a political text giving advice to the Labour government which, being the 'winter of discontent', might actually have had some value! But above all, I was completely obsessed with time, carefully recording the date and time of all sorts of trivial events, covering sheets of paper in a meaningless jumble of figures.

After a home visit by my GP and a psychiatrist, it was agreed I should go to Hellingly Mental Hospital on a voluntary basis, to allow my behaviour to be properly monitored. I must assume I was put under heavy sedation, which forced my mind to relax and get some natural sleep.*8 Nevertheless I can clearly remember, even now, my head being so hot that I used to wander around the ward, trying to find the best place to cool it down.

After a few days I got back to near normal as far as the extreme tension was concerned. I then spent a week in hospital doing next to nothing, a period of staggering boredom when I was unable to do anything, my mind totally exhausted.

There's usually humour to be found in even the direst circumstances. 'Hysterical laughter' is hype much bandied about in plugs for books, plays and even mildly amusing sitcoms. But in my case I can think of few incidents of real uncontrollable, hysterical laughter, and then only during a manic cycle.

An unforgettable hysterical episode took place near the end of my stay in Hellingly. It was a Saturday evening, well past our official bedtime, and, unable to sleep with my head feeling red hot, I got up to stroll around to try to cool it down.

The ward had a central area with two wide corridors leading off from opposite sides, each with locked emergency doors at the end. One side of each corridor, fully glazed, faced across the grounds, which were covered with snow at the time. The temperature outside was below freezing and because of the large glass area, the corridor was the coolest place I could find.

I stood at the end of one corridor for some minutes, but still felt the need for further cooling. I managed to lift up one sash window about six inches, but wooden stops preventing further opening, presumably to stop suicide attempts.

With head turned flat I managed to squeeze it through the gap and for ten minutes enjoyed the wonderful relief from the heat, as the freezing outside air cooled my head right down. Then, realising it was going numb, I reluctantly wriggled it back inside.

As my head quickly warmed up it was comfortable for a few seconds as equilibrium was reached, but the temperature continued to climb into an area of intense distress. My head felt so hot that I went into a state of panic, thinking it was actually, physically on fire.

I looked around, desperate for help. Through the fog of fright and blinding tension, I noticed a fire alarm breakglass right opposite me. I lurched frantically across the corridor, elbow pointing in front of me, and smashed the glass, to my immense relief.

The shock of this violent action, with the immediate ringing of alarm bells throughout the hospital complex, seemed to bring me back to relative sanity. I stood bemused, awaiting the staff response to what, at two o'clock in the morning, they knew had to be a real emergency.

Within a minute there were running footsteps and a kerfuffle on the stairs outside the emergency door. A key was thrust into the lock but it wouldn't open and swearwords bounced around as they struggled — fought, even — to get in. Eventually they got it open and six people, overcoats over nightwear, raced down the corridor into the main area.

Awaiting my own rescue, there was plenty of action as patients were wrapped in blankets and led to safety. The bedridden were wheeled out and then, after several minutes' disciplined teamwork, everything went quiet.

I stood there calmly, until it dawned on me that the person who'd set off the alarm was the only one they'd missed — out of some 300 patients! The sheer irony of this hit me and I dissolved into unstoppable, hysterical laughter. For minutes it went on, tears ran down my face and I was obliged to double up to relieve aching stomach muscles — I could feel the bruising for days afterwards — as the laughter went on and on.

On sober reflection, this story is not that funny and only seemed so because of my state of mind. But, as well as the therapeutic value, it taught me an invaluable lesson: physically cooling the head can give welcome temporary relief from stress, but it's not a permanent solution. And over-cooling, like shaking a bottle of fizz, is clearly not to be recommended. As the saying goes, 'what goes up, must come down'; or more specifically, 'what goes down fast, comes up fast'.

After leaving hospital, I was off work for two months, mainly resting and reading at home. Carol gave me odd jobs to do around the house, which she said I carried out like a robot.

Any bounce or sparkle I possessed had evaporated and I was quiet and subdued, apparently still in a state of shock. My brain operated incredibly slowly, as if mired in treacle, taking seconds to register the simplest comment. I found it exhausting to converse for more than a few minutes, and for some weeks couldn't face the prospect of meeting people socially.

My confidence dipped and I felt slightly self-conscious when talking to strangers —- did they know about this episode, and if so, what did they think? But mostly, the limited capacity of my mind was occupied with mundane tasks and I had little time to ponder the future.

Day to day I could sense my brain toughening and speeding up, bringing my personality back with it. A real test of my recovery was meeting a group of old cricketing pals in the hectic atmosphere of a crowded pub. These were friends with whom I'd so much enjoyed trading insults and quick-fire repartee over the years.

On the occasion I felt nervous and shy, like the embarrassment of joining a swish party, knowingly having egg on the face. By accident or design, my pals did the right thing; they greeted me as if I'd come back from a long holiday, speaking quietly and slowly. As they filled me in with the gossip, I could feel my mind strengthening and quickening, confidence growing.

After the breakdown

Having got back to near normal and resumed work, I began reflecting on the breakdown; in particular, trying to figure out why it had happened. My main point of annoyance was my failure to give even cursory consideration to my mental health; I'd simply bowled along doing anything required, at any pace, in any circumstances, without the slightest thought of over-stretching myself.

Secondly, the possible stressors mentioned before - my mother-in-law's death, and my role as a company director - I decided were only minor, temporary factors in a lifestyle which had remained unchanged for many years prior to the breakdown. There appeared to be no obvious explanation, other than a steady build-up of tension which had come to a head, with shattering effect.

The residue of feelings and changes in my thinking can easily be described. Consideration of my mental health has since been ever present, perhaps even obsessively so. I have felt obliged (wrongly?) to duck and dive continually to avoid getting myself in the same state again.

Far and away the most powerful incentive for this avoidance has been the sheer, unadulterated fear of losing control of my mind again. My only previous experience, which I had always taken for granted, was of my mind functioning rationally and logically.*9 Then and now, I simply can't imagine what life would be like, or whether it would be worth living, without this basic faculty.

No doubt the technical definition of madness is quite complex and strict lines cannot be drawn, but over the months following the event I developed my own simplistic criteria. If my thoughts, however intense, delusive and irrational, did not alter my physical actions in a noticeable way, then I was sane. Once my irrational thought became so powerful it affected my physical actions and/or speech, then I was 'over the top' and into madness.

I've graded in my mind the intensity of the many manic episodes I've been through since on a 1 to 10 basis. Going through an 8 or 9 has been frightening, hovering just below the brink, but these I've considered tolerable and gritted my teeth to get through them. But by my definition, above 10 is into the maelstrom of madness and something I've always fought against tenaciously.

To better equip myself for the immediate post-breakdown period, a number of counselling sessions with psychiatric professionals were arranged. To be brutally honest, I feel I learnt little from most of them. Everyone was well intentioned, but most of the advice seemed so generalised and vague I didn't see how it could provide any practical help for me.

Having said that, I must put my hand up and admit to a degree of arrogance in my approach to counselling of this kind. I've always been much impressed by the saying, 'God helps those who help themselves.' Similarly, I've always felt that the only person who can really unravel the nitty-gritty of the workings of my mind, is me.

Surely, I reasoned, a half-hour session with a stranger, however skilled in the psychiatric field, is not going to teach him much more than the mental equivalent of my name and address. My approach therefore to these sessions was a touch cynical and negative, but didn't stop me from listening to what was said. I thought that even if I could pick up just one piece of advice, it might add to my understanding of what had happened and how a recurrence could be avoided.

Memories of those counselling sessions are vague now, but certain things have stuck in my mind. I was particularly annoyed with one chap, who was determined to uncover an unhealthy relationship with my mother, grilling me the whole session on this one subject. When he finished I felt quite exhausted, as if I'd been aggressively cross-examined in a court of law.

Another session was with a chap with sweater, corduroys, straggly beard and so on, virtually my (prejudiced) image of someone woolly and vague. True to expectation, he waffled on in a whispered monotone, only occasionally bringing me into the dialogue. When we finished, I realised I'd not only learnt nothing, I'd understood virtually nothing either!

By far the most useful treatment was that arranged with a relaxation therapist at the Burnt Mill Clinic in Uckfield. Each session, on a one-to-one basis, was given by a chap about my age, who had a practical, no-nonsense approach to the subject. He taught me the process of relaxing mind and body, and gave me an audio tape to play at home. This I used a lot and found very useful for some years. I don't exercise so formally now but I still use the ideas when I want to try and 'bring myself down', or take a nap.

A small point I remember about that chap was that he always called me 'Fred'. At some stage in each session I would politely correct him, and for a few minutes 'Dick' would be bandied about. Then he would regress to 'Fred' again. It's a small point, but it gave the impression that he was on auto-pilot, destroying any illusion of treatment tailored to the individual.

The 1980s

By the time I'd completed my convalescence and gone back to work, I was confident I'd been through a 'one-off' breakdown, and that everything would return to normal. There'd been no mention from any source of manic depression or mania. I was also unaware of the possibility that irreversible biochemical changes can take place in the brain during a breakdown.

About three months after starting back at work I experienced my first manic episode. I had no idea what was going on except that my head felt hot and I had difficulty going to sleep. I saw my GP who prescribed tranquillisers and, having taken the maximum dose, I returned to near normal after a few days.

I assumed all this was like an 'after-shock' from an earthquake, and would diminish in intensity and eventually disappear. Being a fairly patient soul, I didn't worry too much, and was prepared to put up with it provided I reached my objective of pre-breakdown normality.

Apart from the counselling I'd received, I was only prepared for my post-breakdown life with the relaxation technique, plus a succession of prescription tranquillisers: Mogadon — which gave me a thumping hangover in the morning — Largactil and Stelazine.

It was left to my discretion to take up to three a pills day, something I avoided initially for several reasons. My aversion to regular pill-swallowing meant I saw no point in taking any when I felt relatively calm. This arrangement — unsatisfactory for a reason described later — had the advantage that it didn't 'zombie down' my personality and allowed me to convince myself I'd not become damaged or over-reliant on pills. In addition, and of considerable practical importance, I had to drive some 15 miles to work each day; taking regular tranquillisers could have caused to become a danger on the roads.

As months turned into years, I realised things weren't going back to square one. I was having manic episodes on a regular basis, on average three a year. Slowly and most reluctantly, I accepted that these episodes were to become a recurring feature of my life. Nevertheless I tried hard —-even desperately — to analyse each episode, looking for a pattern or common features, which would enable me to take evasive action or make lifestyle changes.

I was particularly convinced there had to be a stressful event that acted as the 'trigger' for the next episode, thinking there must be a cause and an effect. It also seemed logical that there had to be a direct relationship between periods of heavy and stressful work and the following manic episode.

All my efforts in this direction were thwarted and I was eventually forced to accept there was no way I could anticipate the next episode; they all seemed to take place without warning and at random intervals. I spent much introverted effort trying to figure this out; the fact that I got nowhere was most frustrating and disappointing.

With hindsight, in terms of mental health, the first half of the '80s was the worst period of my life. It seemed that as soon as I got over one manic episode

I was careering uncontrollably towards the next, with no idea how to alter the situation.

'Uncontaminated' by drugs, at least I was able to start compiling my understanding of the manic episode process. Because there are distinct features, usually all happening at once, it took some years before I could distinguish each component. In fact it wasn't till the mid-'90s that I felt I'd finally unravelled the knot and fully understood the individual components. I'm now confident I've learnt as much as I can and have detailed my understanding in a later section.

(I've don't know whether these processes are the same for all mania patients, but the literature I've seen tends to highlight similar aspects.)

When my head felt hot my first reaction was to apply my cold head theory; I would disappear outside somewhere to try and cool down. (Sometimes at work, feeling 'baking' hot and desperate to get relief, I'd drive to the cricket ground, even in mid-winter, and sit alone on a bench, just staring at the empty field.)

At home I'd go for a walk as the tension rose to cool my head down slowly. This process I found invaluable in giving quick, temporary relief and I've used it countless times over the years, and still do today.

I tried to apply the relaxation techniques every day and I was lucky to be able to obtain quiet and restful conditions during each session, bearing in mind we had two boisterous teenagers in the house. Though it may not have relieved the underlying tension, I found it very useful in slowing my mind down, and quite often I would doze off for a few minutes.

But despite my efforts, though I tried to kid myself otherwise, it wasn't getting to the root of the problem. During visits to my GP several different tranquillisers were prescribed, but never was the primary drug treatment for mania - lithium - mentioned.

As I've written before, there's no doubt my work and office conditions were the main source of the stress in my life at that time. It would seem obvious that I should have given up engineering and trained for a new job in a less frenetic, more academic environment. I toyed with this idea at the time but it was easier said than done.

We had teenage children; I was in my forties and the sole bread-winner. We had no spare cash, or easy access to cash, to tide us through the re-training period.

As well as the considerable financial risk, a long period of time - certainly months, perhaps years - could have elapsed before my income would have been restored to its previous level. This in itself would've been a substantial cause of worry. I decided therefore to keep going in my engineering job, drawing some comfort from the saying, 'the devil you know'.

After several years careering through manic episodes, I accepted I'd got an ongoing, perhaps permanent, health problem. I took two decisions, in principle to reduce stress at work, which I hoped would not only achieve this, but also enable me to keep earning a reasonable income up to retirement.

Firstly, I decided not to seek promotion, or allow myself to be promoted, to a job where I was responsible for the management of other people; i.e. a position to 'hire and fire'. Making decisions directly affecting other people's livelihoods are never easy, but in my case I had to remember I might be obliged to make difficult decisions when in an emotionally unstable state. (The downside of this policy of opting out of greater responsibility has been a limitation of my earning power.)

Secondly, there was the matter of my working conditions. Most office workers get moved around as the organisation expands or contracts. About '82 I found myself working with five other engineers in a single room. It was not unduly cramped, but I soon found the continuous activity and noise too much for me. Phones ringing, loud conversations, laughter, people rushing in and out - all effectively destroyed my ability to concentrate.

I decided that to do my job effectively and stay reasonably calm, I had to work in a more peaceful environment. My second principle therefore, was to insist on having my own office, however small it might be. I have managed to achieve this ever since.

From my viewpoint, there were additional advantages to the single office. I can try to adjust the room temperature nearer my preferred colder level for my head. I can grab a few moments of relaxation between spells of mental activity, without colleagues thinking I'm 'nodding off'. Most importantly, I've learnt that to concentrate properly, not only do I need a calm atmosphere, I need to 'relax my mental guard' and be confident my mind won't be brutally 'broken into'.

In the eight years between my first and second breakdowns I had around twenty serious manic episodes, often with minor ones in between. As I careered along through this, I convinced myself I was unravelling the mechanics of the manic episode and (I thought) making necessary adjustments to my lifestyle. But my arrogance, or at least over-confidence, deceived me. Believing I was becoming more proficient at coping with the problem, I wrongly assumed I was tackling the cause of it.

By '87, it was certainly true that I was going through less of the serious, delusive, manic episodes. This persuaded me that, if nothing else, at least I'd always retain control of my mind. And as far as I was concerned, provided I remained sane ('in control'), going through the lesser manic episodes was just a price I had to pay.

My second breakdown

Compared to my first, the second breakdown appeared to be focused on a single intense manic episode. In the weeks leading to the climax, I began waking in the early hours in great distress, my forehead feeling as if clamped with an iron band. One again, visits to my GP resulted in prescriptions for tranquillisers or sleeping pills; clearly the fragility of my mental state had not been recognised. Even a home visit by a doctor earlier on the actual day produced no relevant diagnosis or warning.

In fairness to the medics, so desperate was I to avoid another catastrophe that I tried to fool everyone into thinking there was nothing much wrong with me. My family and close friends could see through this, but it wasn't easy for others to recognise the seriousness of my situation.

May 4th 1987 was undoubtedly the most traumatic day of my life. Even recalling the events more than ten years on makes me feel uncomfortable. Though less aware then of its significance, my head temperature was 'red hot' when I went to bed at my usual time, naively thinking that if the house was totally quiet, I might be able to relax enough to get some proper sleep.

I'd told my son Mark and his cousin — who was staying with us — to keep in their rooms after bedtime and not use the small snooker table we had in the lounge. There was half an hour of silence till they got up, crept into the lounge, shut the door carefully, and started playing. They made no noise, assuming I was asleep or wouldn't hear anything.

As an engineer often involved in acoustic problems, it does seems remarkable that the collision of two small billiard balls could even be heard at such a distance through two closed doors. But to me, with 'enhanced hearing', the clicking of the balls were like miniature explosions in my brain.

Seething with anger, I stormed downstairs and gave the boys an almighty dressing down, the effort of which alone drove my tension level higher. The boys became frightened for both my welfare and their own physical safety, and after discussion with Carol, Mark was sent discreetly next door to make a 999 call for assistance from ambulance and police.

Both services arrived quickly and in the ensuing discussions the need for a doctor was soon agreed. My own GP was off-duty, so an on-call doctor was contacted, and he also arrived promptly.

While all this was going on I was getting more and more irritable; I couldn't understand why we needed all these people and why they were milling about inside my house. (I've since found out that at one point there were - two policemen, a social worker, two ambulancemen, the doctor, two neighbours, my visiting nephew and the four members of my family - in the house!)

I felt (and feel) strongly that 'an Englishman's home is his castle'; and as I'd done nothing wrong there was no reason for the police to be involved. Essentially, all I wanted was everyone to clear off so I could go to bed and try to sleep.

After an interminable period of confusion, it was finally conveyed to me that it was in my best interests to go to Hellingly Hospital, where I could be properly monitored and treated as necessary. Perhaps with the Durham event in mind I refused, saying I wanted to take a suitable sedative and stay at home, confident I'd recover in a few days. (In fact, Carol has since said, and I accept, that she would never have been able to cope with me in the state I was in, while looking after the children as well.)

As pressure increased for me to 'go quietly' I became more resentful and determined to resist going to hospital. I actually got into bed, praying everybody would simply go away, but at this stage the police began to take a more active role. They were getting ready to remove me bodily from my bed and into the ambulance. At that point I gave in, accepted my fate and went quietly, though still furious and resisting anyone touching me.

It must've been around three in the morning when the ambulance finally arrived at Hellingly Hospital. Had I been in normal mood, I'm sure I'd have giggled at the fact that after all the kerfuffle, we couldn't get in! The place was all locked up and more scurrying about was needed before I could be smuggled in through a side door.

Once inside, as expected, I was put to bed and given some sort of 'sleeping pill bomb', which knocked me out for some hours. From then on it was much the same routine as the first time, my head tension level coming down steadily as time passed, agonisingly slowly. Because this time I'd been 'sectioned' for two weeks, the boredom factor seemed much worse.

To this day, I believe the fundamental point missed in this traumatic episode was that of communication.

At that time I knew that 'dangerous, criminal madmen' could be 'sectioned' and incarcerated for the safety of the community. But I was unaware of the detailed provisions of the 1983 Mental Health Act and the fact that non-violent, non-criminal people such as me could also be 'sectioned' if deemed necessary.

My feelings on leaving hospital were similar to those after my first breakdown, but more intense. The superficial embarrassment and loss of self-confidence lasted a few weeks, but much more dominant was the feeling of shock and disbelief. It was shattering to realise all the efforts I'd made to understand and cope with the problem over the previous years had achieved nothing.

When I'd got my mind back to near normal I started to analyse fairly rationally what had gone wrong this time. It took no great thought to realise the problem was beyond me, and I had to get assistance to avoid careering into another breakdown a few years further on.

Even now I can recall the feeling of immense relief when my doctor told me I had a long-term mental health 'problem'. I can't recall precisely whether 'mania' or 'manic depressive' were used, but it felt as if a great burden had been lifted from my shoulders. At least I had a better insight of where I stood and could try to understand the illness through other people's experiences; presumably, I'd be able to get ongoing practical help and advice.

When it was recommended that I start a regular course of lithium carbonate I accepted instantly, with not a thought for my aversion to pill-taking. My feelings of personal defeat swamped any doubts I might have had in going down this road. Decision made; but after further reflection niggling fears were much alleviated by the fact that lithium is an inorganic salt and non-addictive. (My initial dose was 1000mg per day, reduced after eighteen months to 800mg.)

As before, I set off back to work with a prescription for a tranquilliser (Pimozide) to enable me to calm down and get sleep when over-tense or in a manic episode. In the first months, perhaps being over-cautious, I used these more than strictly necessary until I was literally stopped dead in my tracks.

Driving to work one morning, I was too slow joining the main road from a side turning and caused an accident, knocking a young motorcyclist off his bike. Though unhurt myself, there was the full emergency situation with police and ambulance, all of which left me 'shaking like a leaf'. Recovering from the immediate shock, I was immensely relieved, to put it mildly, to learn a few hours later the youngster had suffered only superficial cuts and bruises.

I was charged with driving with 'undue care and attention', although technically it could have been the more serious offence of 'driving under the influence of drink or drugs'. In any event, the hard lesson for me was that I couldn't risk taking regular tranquillisers and drive. And because I had no other practical means of getting to work, it meant I could only use the drug over weekends or on a very occasional basis.

There was however a distinct advantage of this arrangement, in that it allowed me to make a clearer assessment of my stress level and its associated head temperature. (Most of the tranquillisers I'd taken before made my head feel mildly warm and fuzzy, which made it more difficult to read the warning signs when I became over-stressed.)

For the first year taking lithium I was concerned about the possibility of side-effects, but forgot these worries as nothing untoward seemed to happen; the daily dose and three-monthly blood test soon became routine. However, with much longer hindsight, I now believe I've possibly been affected by two of the listed side-effects.

Firstly, I added about a stone to my weight in the first year, and I'm fairly certain this was not due to any obvious change in my eating or exercise habits.

Secondly, I think the function of my thyroid gland has been affected, and after a year or so I was advised to take a daily dose of 100mg of thyroxine. I've also noticed (without any understanding of the technicalities of how lithium affects the metabolism) that I've become acutely sensitive to cold in winter, and heat and direct sunlight in summer.

By the end of the '80s, I'd been taking lithium for three years. It hadn't made any difference to the frequency of manic episodes, but undoubtedly there'd been a significant reduction in intensity. Using my yardstick of 0 to 10 for manic episodes (10 being the brink of 'going over the top', or madness): before lithium I was regularly reaching 8, 9 and 10, but after only 4, 5 and 6. This of course was a huge improvement and my fears of going into the delusive state began to fade.

As a postscript to this section I'd like to make a few comments about Hellingly Mental Hospital, after two visits. Nothing much seemed to have changed between '79 and '87 and for most of the time on each occasion I was in the exhausted, recovery phase, after the peak of the breakdown.

On entering the hospital, my first reaction was that of intense shame and humiliation at being locked in; rather as I presume a first offender feels entering jail. It also struck me as unnecessary because, while some patients in my ward might have been dangerous, nothing I'd ever done suggested I might be likewise.

The air temperature in the main ward must have been around 26 Celsius, necessary perhaps for the older patients. For me, already with high head temperature, this was the worst possible environment. At times the heat seemed absolutely stifling and drove me to wander around searching for the coolest place in the ward.

I don't see why it shouldn't be possible to provide the odd room in the ward with an air temperature around 20 Celsius. This would allow patients who felt so inclined the chance to cool down, although I've always accepted that this gives only temporary, physical relief.

However my most vivid memory of Hellingly, and in a sense my biggest complaint, was that of total, sheer boredom. For most of the time there was nothing I could do which would hold my attention for more than a few seconds, though to be fair, when completely mentally exhausted there was little I was capable of doing; the more strenuous activities were only suitable for those close to recovery.

The hospital had a game room for table tennis and snooker. There was also a TV lounge and reading room. But none of these facilities were of any real use to me in my addled state of mind.

The 'enhanced sound' of colliding snooker balls was too painful for my oversensitive brain, while watching TV, with its rapidly changing images and unbroken noise, was far too active and stressful. Reading was pointless as I couldn't remember a sufficient amount of the preceding text to make the effort worthwhile. All this left me nothing else to do other than stroll around, sit and look at the pictures in a magazine, or try and make polite conversation with another patient.

A vivid memory of the boredom was sitting on my bed, watching the hands of the clock move round, waiting for the time of the next visit by Carol or other friends to arrive. Talking quietly with visitors was the one part of the day when I could communicate at my pace and feel I was back in the real world.

Two things come to mind which I could have handled and might have alleviated my boredom. A large tropical fish tank; the slow moving, colourful images would have just kept my mind ticking over. Alternatively a large screen video, with slow-moving countryside scenes, perhaps with animals and a gentle soundtrack, could also have had the same effect.

I understand Hellingly is no longer used for mental health patients, so perhaps its replacement has got things like this, though I'm not too anxious to find out!

Into the 1990s

The concept of 'stress management' seemed a fancy new idea much in vogue in the '80s. Yet in an amateurish way I had made every effort to avoid doing things I thought might hasten the next manic episode. However, something that increasingly irritated me and seemed grossly unfair, was that not only did I get tensed up by work, but also when I was supposed to be enjoying myself.

An example to illustrate this problem - and which led me towards the solution - was when Carol and I went to a neighbour's party one evening. Nothing much was happening when we arrived - just other couples mostly whispering separately to one other.

Seeing this as pointless, I waded in and kick-started conversations, asking provocative questions or making contentious comments. This got the ball rolling by engendering fighting, sometimes indignant, responses.

My efforts served their purpose, with everyone soon chatting together, but I also realised my temperature had gone 'sky high' with the concentrated mental effort. It stayed that way long after the party finished and attempts to cool myself down had little effect. Even with the maximum Pimozide dose, I couldn't sleep properly for two days and generally had a pretty unpleasant time. The episode left me both depressed and confused.

A week later I had to see my GP over a physical problem. That was soon sorted but as he wrote up his notes he asked, 'everything all right?', meaning of course my mental health. Still uptight about the party, the dam burst and I quickly and colourfully garbled out the story, finishing with how fed up I was that I couldn't even enjoy the odd night out.

When I stopped he looked up and said quietly, 'You must go out, then in, out, then in.' As he said 'out' he stretched his arm straight forward with fingers spread and palm facing me. Saying, 'in', he drew his hand back to his chest with fist clenched.

Instantly I knew exactly what he meant. Had I not been in the hushed confines of a doctor's surgery, I'd have punched the air in delight. Without doubt it was, and remains, by far the single most important piece of advice about mania I've ever received.

I put this idea into action immediately, with dialogue or anything that involved concerted mental activity. By making myself 'take a breather' between bouts of effort, I found my head temperature didn't go too high, enabling me to stay at a steady, cool level.

In the early '90s, after our children had left home, I was able to concentrate much more on my lifestyle and try to arrange things to minimise the mania. But in '91 I was made redundant during a time of deep recession, with no immediate possibility of finding employment. Surprisingly perhaps, in the two years I was out of full time work, I didn't go through any serious manic episodes. Of course the financial worry was considerable and on-going — like a long dull ache in the brain — but I managed to adopt a philosophical view; there was nothing much I could do about it.

Once back to full-time work, I was able to refocus on stress reduction. After some five years taking lithium, I'd built enough confidence to believe I could avoid the more serious manic episodes — of the delusory kind anyway. It was at about this time that an incident occurred which showed what a huge psychological prop the drug had become.

Carol and I went away for a weekend break, taking just an overnight bag. At my usual pill-taking time I searched my bag but couldn't find them. After much anxious rummaging I finally accepted I'd forgotten them and at that instant, for the first and only time in my life, I had an intense 'flashback'.

All the parts of Hellingly Hospital I'd seen, plus all the patients I'd met, zipped through my mind at great speed. Though it lasted only a few seconds, I stood bemused as my head temperature soared and I started to sweat. It was a stunningly powerful, and quite frightening, experience.

Outside my job I took every opportunity to reduce stress, on the assumption that a quiet, peaceful and orderly existence should reduce the likelihood of manic episodes. Broadly speaking, I determined to live within my income, avoid confrontations or pressurised situations, and tried not to commit myself to a tight deadline in anything I undertook.

In my job, I'd developed strategies over the years to protect myself: keeping a list of work to be done, writing notes to convey information to colleagues, clearly delineating my specific responsibilities, concentrating on one job at a time, and above all, 'binning the junk'. By that I mean, clearing my mind of the details of a particular project as soon as it's finished. I've got this to such a fine art now that I usually can't remember much about a job I've finished even a day later.

The other aspect of my life which started to assume greater importance was sleep: not only have I steadily placed greater attention on the quantity and quality of sleep, but, because I'm not 'contaminated' by sedatives or tranquillisers, monitoring my sleep pattern gives me a good indication of my general state of mind.

I can't be quite sure that a deterioration in my sleep quality forewarns me of a manic episode, but it certainly tells me when I'm going through one and, importantly, when the cycle's completed. Nowadays I prepare carefully for bed - a bit like a jumbo jet pilot before take-off! - to ensure I have the optimum conditions for a peaceful, untroubled night.

An entirely new revelation in the early '90s was the discovery of the limits of my ability to concentrate continuously, and my mental stamina generally. In a haphazard way, one incident after another provided warnings as to what I could and couldn't undertake without developing a hypertense 'hot head' state; they dramatically underlined my GP's advice about the key importance of rationing continuous concentration.

The first episode that modified my thinking was driving a car, which of course involves continuous concentration. I found I could drive comfortably for no more than 90 minutes at speeds up to 60 mph. If I went above that speed, the greater concentration needed caused a steady rise in head temperature.

Another lesson on driving was when Carol and I decided to visit our daughter in Plymouth, a 260 mile journey. Leaving at midday, we intended to split the drive into three sections, with breaks in between; I would do the first and last and Carol the middle.

Everything went to plan till it came to Carol's turn; she didn't feel too well, so I drove all the way. We made extra stops and kept our speed down, but in spite of this I was amazed at what happened when we arrived.

Getting out of the car, I was introduced to someone and immediately made a silly remark, then started giggling. It seemed the pent-up tension had been released, my temperature had shot up, and I'd gone into a euphoric, light-headed state, full of cheeky chat which lasted till the next day.

Another embarrassing lesson was when I applied for a job in '92. At the interview, for the first time in my life I had to take aptitude tests. The first lasted ten minutes, the second twenty, and we had to answer as many questions as we could in the time.

I knew I would be asking for trouble by attempting these and sure enough, my head temperature shot up rapidly. By the time we'd finished it was red hot and I was soon giggling and making stupid remarks.

The situation might have been retrieved for the formal interview but —-Murphy's law — mine was the first! With no intervening period to cool down, I said some pretty silly things, and predictably, was not asked to return for the final interview.

Learning from these incidents, it seemed intense concentration for a short period, or mild concentration for a long period, could have the same effect. It encouraged me to develop some ground rules to minimise the problem.

When I go to a party, or any occasion which might be noisy and require continuous mental activity, I try to plan an escape route. I look for somewhere outside, preferably quiet, where I can go for a walk or just sit alone for a few minutes, to allow my head to cool down. By doing this (several times if necessary) I can avoid going up into that state of 'irreversible' tension which destroys my sleeping pattern and may take days to return to normal.

My friends soon learnt about my strategy and nothing more needed to be said, but going to the cinema, theatre or any indoor public performance is another matter. Obviously I could get up and walk out if the pressure's too great, but it's not as simple as that.

If I were to walk out of a theatre, it may be a nuisance to others and that has an inhibiting effect. Also, anyone with me might be concerned for my welfare and feel obliged to follow. As far as the cinema or discos are concerned, I'm simply frightened about subjecting myself to (what I'm told!) is the normal shattering sound level.

By the mid-90s I was confident I'd figured out my capacity — or lack thereof! — for continuous concentration and rapid mental activity. This has enabled me to 'duck and dive' at work and social events since then, to keep my head cool and avoid getting over-tense. I also think — or rather, hope — that avoiding 'over-heating' may delay or reduce the intensity of the next manic episode.

Having taken lithium for ten years I decided to see the local psychiatrist to run through my current thinking and see if I could pick up any useful tips on mania. 'Disappointingly' he seemed to agree with most of what I said, so I gleaned nothing to alter my approach to the problem.

He did however recommend I take carbamazepine to enhance(?) the effect of lithium. This I've done with a daily dose of 200mg since November '97. I can't really say I've noticed any difference, but I understand there's a sedative effect that may have improved my sleeping.

At this point I decided to write up my experiences of mania while starting a contemporaneous diary from the beginning of '98, which continues below.

In the later appendices my 'thinking' about various aspects of mania are spelt out, particularly my understanding of the process of the manic episode.

Diary from 1998

At the start of the year I was calm and remained so till mid-February, when I went through a minor episode, the cycle being completed in about a week. It was brought about by a work problem which I thought would be much worse than actually transpired. In a sense my pessimism created this episode.

On the 27th March my cricket club, St James's Montefiore, held their Centenary Dinner at a hotel in Hove. Playing cricket over 35 years has been the greatest source of fun to me and I have a deep sentimental attachment to the Club. When asked to be Toastmaster I readily accepted, though I knew this would drive my adrenaline sky high.

By tradition the four speakers and Toastmaster try to be funny, with jokes and anecdotes focused on the local cricket scene. As well as running the show in light-hearted style, my task was to make witty introductions to each speaker.

I worked hard on my material for weeks before, well aware that after-dinner speaking in humorous vein is far more difficult than it may appear. In the days before the Dinner I became grimly focused on my role, and recognised I was entering a manic cycle.

As usual, everything went 'alright on the night', regarded as a success by all. I was able to read symptoms of the manic episode, the 'staring effect' being prominent. Fortunately, I remembered to allow for the 'speeding up' effect and took advice from others before calling the next toast or speaker. This ensured the Dinner didn't finish 45 minutes earlier than usual!

In early March I started work on probably the largest air conditioning equipment project of its type in the world, with packaged plant valued into millions. My role was that of co-ordinator of the bid: establishing the detailed design, building up cost estimates and preparing the multiple quotations necessary.

I'd done this sort of thing often before, but not at the pace demanded by current conditions, everything being governed by the site programme. To save time, I learnt the specification by heart and retained much other data in my head.

With so much at stake I was also subject to constant pressure from management and sales staff, this situation continuing into early August when the contract was finally won. By then I had become aware of my growing mental exhaustion, loss of humour, and focus on this one subject; that I was 'hanging on with clenched teeth'.

On August 14th I was told I'd completed my part of the project and would have no further executive role. This triggered an immediate flood of relief, similar to the effect after the peak of a manic episode. Within hours it seemed I was 'binning the junk', clearing out all the surplus data, relaxing to start the climb back to full mental strength.

To my surprise, my sleeping pattern, interrupted for some weeks, remained irregular right into early October. It seems I'd over-stretched my capacity for long term mental stamina, and though the symptoms were mild around the peak, I'd been through a kind of long, flat manic cycle lasting about seven months.

From then on, remarkably perhaps, no further problems; fingers crossed!

1999

My New Year's resolution, health-wise, was to try and put all my introverted thoughts about mania to the back of my mind. The rough draft for 'Living with mania' had been written so there was no point in becoming too obsessed with the subject (such obsession probably being counter-productive).

In a day-to-day sense I've decided to be guided by just two of the various aspects of mania I've talked about and tackle the others as they occur. The first is the 'hot head' feeling; when this occurs I'll take whatever action I can to reduce temperature. The second - which is of increasing importance to me - is the monitoring of my state of mind by the quality of my sleep.

In February I lost control when talking to a client on the phone at work. The man was an unprincipled liar and I 'blew up' and couldn't stop myself becoming overly heated. Others soon took over and resolved the situation, but the stress destroyed my sleeping pattern for days.

Ironically, this incident coincided with reports in the media that the long-running debate between psychiatrists on this subject had finally been resolved. *10

My daughter's wedding day was June 5th. With all the organisation being done by others, my sole task was my speech as father of the bride. I've done a fair amount of public speaking so wasn't unduly worried about it, but naturally I was determined to do my level best for this unique occasion.

Nevertheless, subconscious worries about the event gave me broken nights' sleep for about a month before, and in the three days prior to the big day, I recognised from my speech and writing the symptoms of a minor manic episode.

My usual technique for a speech is to list 'bullet points' and then play it off the cuff. But as a precaution for this event, I typed the speech out, word for word, in case I dried up.

On the day this proved a life-saver; I was so hot-headed and high with adrenaline I couldn't remember anything at all and had to rely totally on my notes. I literally staggered outside to cool down immediately afterwards and was disappointed to find it was a warm, muggy evening.

I didn't seem to go through the typical after-peak part of a manic episode but got back to normal fairly quickly. My sleeping pattern returned within about three or four days.

The company I'd been working for became very short of work by mid-summer. Though I wasn't responsible for bringing in enquiries, I felt it was my duty to be available at any time to process those received and put in the most competitive bid. Though not a direct worry, this had played on my mind. On October 15th I was asked by the company's management to reduce my hours by 20%. Surprisingly, this had a positive effect; it was as if a switch had been thrown, relieving stress by 'lifting my nose from the grindstone'.

Fortunately, I can now live with the reduced income without too much difficulty or change of lifestyle. It seems I've become more relaxed in the general sense, my sleeping pattern has improved, and I've enjoyed a high percentage of trouble-free nights since then.

So, into the new millennium, essentially in (relatively) good mental order, ready to face the challenges ahead, etc., etc.!

2000

In mid-January I made an appointment to see the local community psychiatrist, principally to try to find out what I could expect to happen, mania-wise, as I get older. He had made a casual remark some time ago that the problem tends to get worse with age. This had not exactly worried me, but it was not an exciting prospect.

I believe by altering my lifestyle and creeping along carefully, I've reduced the intensity and number of manic episodes over the past few years. And I've got to a point where I can usually relate each episode to a specific stressful event. Generally, my confidence in my ability to live with mania has grown such that, on a day-to-day basis, the subject's no longer at the front of my mind.

The discussion we had was of an upbeat tone and he soon said (as he usually does!) that I knew much more about the mechanics of mania than he did. Whether he makes this statement as the truth, gentle flattery, or an obvious attempt to boost morale, I'm not sure. But it certainly took the sting out of my questions and, to some extent, negated the point of the interview.

When I pinned him down on the age issue, after a lengthy discussion it was clear he had no precise information on this subject. Understandably perhaps, there are no comparative records, and a multitude of variables for every patient.

However, he would not budge from his general opinion that mania intensified with age which, in the absence of any other reason, could obviously be attributed to the ageing process.

Note: Though light-hearted and amicable, this meeting did have considerable psychological importance for me. I came away dispirited and disappointed; if the psychiatrist's views were right it was clear I'd never be able to relax my guard, whatever confidence I'd developed in coping with mania. And though not spelt out as such, it seemed to me that for the rest of my days I'd have to run faster in order to stand still.

Also, as I've done for years, I'll have to continue assessing everything I want to do, or am asked to do, to determine its likely affect on me. The only possible long-term strategy seemed to be to continue applying all my experience of mania to minimise the distress caused.

On January 27th I was due to go to a site meeting in Oxford. As luck would have it, a train strike had been called for that day and it looked as if I'd have to drive the 80-odd miles each way. In the depth of winter, this prospect much worried me, particularly as I had to go on my own.

The problem was solved when a route was found using another train company and I made the trip without further ado. This was an example of my pessimism amplifying my worries about mania; the anticipated problems giving me much unnecessary concern. So this pointless worry generated stress and affected my sleep for several days before and after the event.

I've already mentioned the annual dinner of my cricket club, St James's Montefiore. That year it was held at the end of March in the pavilion of the County Ground, Hove.

There are so many people there I don't see that often now, and the intensity of the chat - coupled with the steadily rising room temperature - meant I had to cool myself down before the speeches started. The location is ideal for this as I could wander outside and stroll round the outfield.

Unfortunately, I bumped into another chap doing likewise, who suffers from schizophrenia so severe he can work only infrequently. I felt obliged to talk to him and offer what sympathy and ideas I could, but it meant I wasn't getting my break. I found the effort becoming quite distressing and, in the end, made an excuse and hurried off, in near darkness, to another part of the ground.

With great relief I drank in the cool air and quiet. Suddenly I was shocked to feel a hand on my shoulder: it was another old pal also walking round the ground. Once again I had to chat for a bit before I could get away.

By the time I got a break my brain felt bruised and I was mentally exhausted. Stupidly, the delay meant I missed the speeches and much of the fun of the occasion.

This episode emphasised once again my need to take a 'breather' at increasingly frequent intervals at any function involving highly stimulating mental activity. For a function to arouse such stimulation does not necessarily require my being involved; just being on the receiving end can be enough to get my head temperature rising.

In April my wife Carol became caught up in the most serious and worrying incident of our entire married life. She was in Ashdown Forest one day with others carers from Grove Park School and a group of children with multiple learning difficulties.

The boy she was responsible for was wearing a wrist restraint to stop him running away, but wasn't responding to any instructions, so had to be gently pulled along. A man sitting in his car watching decided her action amounted to mis-treatment and wrote a colourful letter to the school, copied to the Social Services Department.

A full police investigation was triggered, with a detective knocking at our door, unannounced, to conduct a tape-recorded interview with Carol about the incident. For nearly a month we heard no more from officialdom about the matter, during which time Carol became quite frantic with worry and seriously depressed. Eventually the matter was cleared up and Carol fully exonerated.

For my part, I did whatever I could to help: made phone calls, wrote letters, all the while trying to keep Carol on an even keel. As a secondary consideration, I assumed from the outset that the stress would initiate a major manic episode at some point. In fact, when Carol received the final clearance, naturally I experienced a tremendous surge of relief, but none of the usual manic symptoms.

My sleeping pattern had been disturbed for several weeks and I usually got up once a night, though this was not that unusual. But there was one aspect of my sleep which I can't remember happening before. Around the height of the trauma I was waking after about two hours, with a start, and felt as if my head was nailed to the pillow. It would take five to ten seconds before I could summon strength to co-ordinate mind and body to lift it; a most weird sensation.

To summarise: this episode was the first time it had been imperative to focus my mind continuously on someone else, rather than my own introverted self. I'm not clear how to interpret the fact that I'd got through this test with no suggestion of a manic episode.

At the end of August I held a party at the cricket ground to celebrate my 60th birthday. With over 50 old friends present, it was a most enjoyable evening but, as the centre of attention, I was continuously engaged in chat. One reason I'd chosen the venue was the outfield; by strolling round on my own several times, I managed to keep my head cool.

In October, Carol and I, with two friends, went on a short holiday to Spain. Because we'd decided not to try and do too much I had no mental problems, but I realised afterwards that the travelling aspect was in itself tiring. For example, just waiting at an airport among a sea of continuously moving people, I found quite exhausting.

I got through it alright but it certainly didn't whet my appetite for more foreign travel.

Most Saturdays I go for a walk round Lewes golf course with regular players and friends. It's good exercise and there are spectacular views across the downs. In winter, being outside for 3 or 4 hours can be quite chilling, so on return to the clubhouse my head would be very cold. I noticed that after half an hour in the warm room my head temperature rose right up, making it necessary to go outside to cool down again.

One day in October it dawned on me I was over-cooling my head, so for the first time ever I've taken to wearing a baseball cap in these conditions. It seemed to work immediately; my head being only warmish in the clubhouse after the walk.

At the end of October I was called by my doctor, who advised me my blood lithium content had risen above the danger level. She recommended I reduce the dose from 800 to 600mg per day and have another blood test early in the New Year. This was the first time my dosage had been changed for over ten years.

On Friday, December 8th I attended a dinner with old cricket friends above a pub in Hove. These were people I'd known since the '60s. It was a smallish room and the talk was quite animated, so yet again, within an hour I had to go outside to cool down. Once more, I was disappointed by this problem occurring in such otherwise pleasant and relaxed circumstances.

The following evening we went out in a foursome to an Indian restaurant. Again my head soon got very hot and I had to go outside more than once. I remember now it also seemed as if everyone was rushing about and talking loudly, which I should have recognised as a symptom of an approaching episode.

On Wednesday 13th I was asked to do a 'panic' job at work: it had to be completed by the following morning. It seemed everyone was rushing around the office and, with hindsight, I think that period was around the climax of a minor manic episode. I'd been through this one — only a few days — without reading any of the usual symptoms on the run-up, and it was all over as quickly as it started.

I felt obliged to attend the firm's annual Christmas lunch on Friday 22nd December. It's no exaggeration to say that I was not looking forward to the event, as I fully expected the hot head effect to reoccur.

As a calculated policy to help me cope, I bagged a seat at the end of a table, as far as possible from the centre of activity. And crucially, I allowed the conversation to come to me and simply responded in a steady, low key way.

. In other words, I listened to and enjoyed other people's chat but made no effort to start conversations, tell stories or engage in repartee. Though pretty unsociable and boring for others, the experiment worked perfectly, aided perhaps by a cool room temperature.

This little victory certainly cheered me for Christmas and over that period I enjoyed as good a sleeping pattern as at any time earlier in the year.

2001

In April my main employers moved their factory from Burgess Hill to Partridge Green in West Sussex. As this meant an additional 10 miles each way on my journey to work, I made an agreement that I would work about half the time from home.

Immediately, I found the effect of working at home — for the first time — dramatically reduced my stress level.   Shielded from 'panic' calls, I was able to concentrate on the task in hand in peace and quiet. By itself, this arrangement gave me a new lease of life, allowing me to hope the next manic episode had been pushed further over the horizon.

Running alongside this positive development was a dispute with my employer, the details of which are too complex to detail here.   Normally if I fall out with someone I try to sort out the problem, then walk away if that's not possible.

This dispute caused me intense anger; I felt I was being treated contemptuously and promises had been broken.   But because I had few other employment options at this stage of my life, I was obliged to 'grin and bear it'.

My anger was such that I'm sure it induced a minor manic episode lasting for two to three months during the summer.   Trapped as I was, I forced myself to look at the positive aspects of my working life, and downgrade the strength of my feelings on the issue. The dispute remains unresolved and, though I've had to bite my lip on many occasions, I've felt it prudent to bottle up my true feelings at this stage of my working life.

The second event occurred at the end of September and was of particular interest to me. Over more than twenty years coping with mania I've always thought that work stresses must be the prime cause of most manic episodes I've had. Yet they've never seemed to coincide precisely in time with a major work problem, or else there have been other contributory factors. For the first time however, I'm certain that this specific episode was caused solely by the pressures of a particular project, which had to be completed to a very tight deadline. Before I started, all my other peripheral activities were running smoothly, my sleeping pattern was good and I was generally, 'cool, calm and collected'.

I had about two weeks to submit the bid for a prestigious project. Things started to get fraught immediately: the client made fundamental design changes and re-issued basic requirements, the specification was vague, I had to await clarification on certain points, there were drastic space limitations imposed and the sound level limits and factory testing requirements were 'horrendous'.

On top of that, the project was for the client's own new office building; everyone involved therefore was extremely nervous about making mistakes. Also, one sensed, there was much interdepartmental 'leaning over of shoulders' to complicate matters further.

In the last week I knew I was going into a manic episode; all the usual symptoms were developing. But as soon as the job was finished, I quickly peaked into the recovery phase and I was back to normal within days.

Footnotes for 2001:
Working from home has been a great boon and illustrated what I'm now certain has been one of the root causes of my problems over the years. Put simply: my brain is not capable of handling the complexities of my job, in poor working conditions and to a deadline, without screwing my mind up into a manic condition.

The year also highlighted another point I'd never given any thought to previously. Since I've been working from home I've had three clear days off and been able to fully relax my mind. This is fine but it means that, come Monday morning, when I'm thrown back into the hurly-burly of the office, I've found my brain takes some time to raise its tempo, or get 'up to speed'.

That doesn't matter as such, but if I push myself too fast I can feel my head temperature rise rapidly and this is like (as I've described elsewhere) a minor 'punch' to the brain. To avoid this situation, I've found it necessary to try and warm up my mind somehow before it's hit by the office environment. *11

2002

In late February I went through a very mild manic episode which I'm confident was entirely work related.

Things went along smoothly until an incident in May, which I believe was the most dramatic demonstration to date, of my need to avoid continuous mental effort.

For some years I've made it a rule that I always take a half hour break at lunchtime, when I sit quietly and read while having a sandwich. Invitations to go round the pub for a quick drink are always turned down. This quiet period provides the essential relaxation my brain seems to need after a morning's work.

On May 2nd I was working at home when my son Mark arrived to do a few odd jobs around the house. I had a fairly heavy workload that day, with deadlines to meet by the evening, so I kept going till my usual lunch break while he got on with the jobs. During lunch, as I was obviously pleased to see Mark, we sat in the lounge with a sandwich and had a continuous and slightly animated chat.

I felt one or two twinges, and a slight bruised feeling around the temples, but when my head started to get noticeably 'hot' it was time to get back to work. This became more of a struggle as the afternoon wore on, but I felt obliged to keep going. My ability to concentrate became impaired and likewise I was unable to think too fast.

In the evening I found it too noisy and active to watch television, so I wandered about the house feeling quite unable to do anything. But after a near normal night's sleep I expected to be fully fit by the morning. To my surprise I felt dreadful all day.

I find it most difficult to describe the sensation, other than feeling bruised, addled and distressed in the head; as if somehow my brain had been stirred up. It was impossible to concentrate for more than a minute or two, any sudden noise made me physically jump, and I simply wanted to shut the world off and out completely.

Again, I kept to my usual routine in the evening and again, I didn't know what to do. In the end I sat in a darkened room, playing gentle music at low volume till bed-time. I had a reasonable night's sleep and on Saturday felt much better.

The painful lesson from this episode appeared obvious; I had broken one of my own 'golden rules'. I had allowed myself to get carried away, enjoying chatting to my son, when it was time to take a break. I was shocked by the intensity of the distress I subsequently went through, making me determined to avoid the same mistake again.

On June 22nd I experienced another clear-cut incident of the physical pain induced by over-stretching my mind.

I'd had a couple of easy days before the Saturday and decided to go down to my beloved cricket ground at Ditchling. My idea was to watch the game from about 4 o'clock and possibly meet up with a few old chums.

When I got there I felt as cool and relaxed mentally as I can be at this stage of my life. I wandered around, chatted a bit, then met up with two pals with whom I started playing cricket over 40 years ago.

Soon, the reminiscences stated to flow, then a bit of sharp repartee, and I could feel my head getting hot. Deciding this was a price worth paying for some verbal fun, I kept going a bit longer till I became aware of a sharp pain developing across my forehead.

I stopped the chat immediately, made an excuse, and wandered outside on my own to cool down. The pain developed to a quite intense level then started to ease off. I stayed for another twenty minutes talking quietly on a one-to-one basis, then drove home.

By the time I got home after the half-hour drive, around 8 o'clock, the pain had gone, though my head still felt hot. By keeping cool, reading and listening to music for the rest of the evening, I was back to square one by the time I went to bed.

During the rest of the year, I didn't go through anything that, by my definition, I would call a manic episode. There had been several occasions at work when I'd got a bit panicky and over-heated about something, but in each case I got things back to normal within a few hours.

Footnote to 2002:

The final few months of the year had seen a fundamental shift in my approach to mania. After years of ducking and diving trying to avoid bringing on manic episodes, I felt it was time to put these precautions and defensive reactions on the back burner to some extent. My priority from then on would seem to be to avoid over-tiredness, and particularly, to not push myself into a state of mental exhaustion.

To assist this, I refused to take on what we call 'panic' estimates at work. This is when a client wants certain design details and prices within hours rather than days. These jobs necessarily involve a period of intense mental activity and I've told my colleagues I'm simply too old to stretch myself anymore.

I've noticed I can feel the tiredness setting in as I get to the end of my working week. As an engineer, I use a calculator every few minutes and this gives me a ready indicator of my mental state. As I start to get too tired my ability to operate this simple gadget slows noticeably and if I go too far, my calculations become laboured. Ultimately, without it, I'm quite literally unable to add two and two together.

2003

No problems in the first two months; I stuck to my four day week and didn't allow myself to get wound up over any job.

On Wednesday, March 5th I went to a pub with an old friend immediately after a day at the Partridge Green factory. We chatted for about an hour and a half, at the end of which I felt exhausted. I didn't sleep well.

On the Thursday, I worked from home all day, with few interruptions. But somehow, unwittingly, I must've over-stretched myself. The next day I felt hot and muzzy and was unable to concentrate for more than a minute or two.

In the evening we had to go out for a long-standing dinner date with two old friends. Aware I could get into greater trouble, I went outside regularly to cool down and reduced my normal level of contributions to the chat. (They must've wondered about the state of my bladder!)

On Saturday I didn't feel too well (though I've felt worse) and so stayed at home doing nothing to test my mind. Sunday was better, but the problem didn't really clear up till late afternoon. This incident shocked me. It made me realise how low my threshold of exhaustion had become, and how careful I've got to be in future to ensure I don't concentrate or engage in continuous mental activity for too long. I now keep this in mind all the time as a matter of priority.

The weather during June, July and August was continuously hot, with various records being broken. Sleeping upstairs with the heat trapped under the roof meant that most nights the room temperature was between 25 and 30 degrees Celsius. I found this most uncomfortable, waking each morning feeling drunk and drowsy, reminiscent of my experiences long ago of the less agreeable tranquillisers.

In December I was called in to my doctor's surgery for a routine check-up, which of course included a blood pressure test. In the week prior to this I'd been working hard on a complex design project with a tight deadline coinciding roughly with my check-up. The other checks were satisfactory but my blood pressure reading was exceptionally high, so much so that the nurse felt obliged to consult my doctor immediately. I was given various instructions and had further blood pressure readings taken over the next few weeks, at the end of which the pressure was above optimum but not dangerously so.

My doctor prescribed a daily dose of 50mg of Atenolol, a beta-blocker, to be taken until further notice. The principle purpose of this drug, I understand, is to reduce and stabilise blood pressure.

Remarkably I noticed from the first day I started taking Atenolol that I didn't experience the 'hot head' feeling at any time, something which seemed almost too good to be true.

2004

This year transpired to be the most trouble-free (from the mental health angle) of any I can remember since my first breakdown.

My working life tailed off into semi-retirement and, although my major client went into liquidation in June, by then I'd conditioned myself to accept that I'd have to dip into my savings to secure an income until drawing my pension from August 2005.

I did in fact do work for other clients but this was sufficiently infrequent that I was able to ensure I didn't get seriously 'wound up' by my work at any time.

For the first time in my life, I'd managed to psychologically de-couple myself from the ingrained, essential drive of having to work hard for my living. For the whole of 2004 therefore, I had no hint of a manic episode.

I also carefully monitored the 'hot head' feeling throughout the year. On no occasion did this occur, even when at one or two social events, I deliberately pressurised the situation by staying for a lengthy period in a hot, noisy room. With increasing confidence, by the middle of the year I'd virtually forgotten that I'd ever had a problem in this area.

In December I went for my routine blood pressure and lithium level tests. My lithium showed an upward trend, consistent with the ageing factor, and I was advised to reduce my daily dose to 400mg, the lowest it's ever been.

My blood pressure level measured around the ideal, leading to a slightly surprised raising of eyebrows, as well as congratulations, by my doctor.

<u>Note</u>: The correlation between blood pressure and my head stress, or temperature, is not something I'd ever previously considered. I'd never read anything about it or received any advice from a medical person since my mania troubles started. My bleak pessimism based on this problem has started to recede and I'm even flirting with the idea of enjoying a few years 'mania-free' retirement!

Appendices

(1) My ideas

After more than 20 years living with and thinking about mania, I've developed my own ideas about the condition and adapted my lifestyle as best I can. Obviously, without medical or psychiatric knowledge I can only go so far in this self-analysis, but nevertheless, it makes things easier for me to have some guidelines for living with the problem.

I now work to the simple basic premise that my brain, in the physical sense at least, is essentially lacking in stamina and relatively over-sensitive to the input of noise, visual images and stress generally.

This has two practical effects: my brain is unable to strike the balance between stress received and stress discharged, successfully achieved by 'normal' people. Over a period, usually months, this leads to a build-up of stress until a manic episode commences. The episode appears to discharge the pent-up stress and when completed, brings things back into balance again.

Secondly, there are restrictions on my ability to concentrate, in terms of continuity and stamina. As well as the usual meaning of concentration I include the unbroken, and usually fast, inflow of data to the brain via sight and sound. And to be expected, I tire quicker mentally than others of my age.

The above theory may be psychiatric nonsense, but it matches my experience and gives me a framework for coping with the problem. Generally, my approach is to protect my brain by minimising stress input, limit data inflow and provide optimum physical conditions for its operation, conscious and unconscious.

My understanding of these stresses and conditions are:

Head temperature. As previously mentioned, the most comfortable air temperature around the head is about 16 Celsius. I believe, in sleeping mode, research suggests the optimum is around 13C.

Without doubt, the quickest and easiest method of relief when I get over-tense or the 'hot head' feeling in any situation, is to physically cool it down. Usually this can't be obtained indoors (without air conditioning!), so I go outside. Over the years I must have done that thousands of times; for a full-scale walk, a stroll round the block, or just standing at the bottom of the garden staring at the fence.

I should add that as well as physical cooling, a period on my own can also release me from the pressures of the other stress inputs I've listed below, at the same time. So it creates a period when I can cool and rest my brain at the same time.

As a consequence to this, I now dislike warm climates, places, or activities that make me physically hot. I've developed a perhaps irrational fear I may be getting too tense and worry the prevailing heat may be masking my ability to monitor my head temperature properly.

An example of this is swimming; as a basic swimmer, the exercise raises my pulse and heart beat as expected. But also, the body is cooled more efficiently by water, while the head is cooled less effectively by air. The immediate and disconcerting sensation I get therefore is that my head is getting hot.

(Without being too pessimistic, a fear I have about advanced old age is to be continuously trapped, by immobility perhaps, in an overheated, noisy inside place.)

Walking. As well as the simplest method of cooling my head, a walk outside has significant other functions. It allows me to take a break from people, televisions, telephones and all other domestic activity and substantially reduce the data inflow to my brain. Also, by putting a distance between any noise or active visual source, I can relax my 'mental guard' against shocks.

For the basic cooling function, with head uncovered, I can cool my forehead down to my comfort zone quite easily. If I'm really 'high', in freezing weather I've sometimes returned home numb with cold, but at least my mind has been slowed and I've won some temporary respite. (I've learnt to watch out for the bounce effect!).

I select my walk depending if I want minimal noise, interesting scenery or the simplest most convenient route. It would seem obvious, living where I do, to get away from traffic noise and go onto the forest, but that's not always practical if it's too muddy.

On balance I prefer a level walk with solid surface and tend to go a similar route most times. This avoids the distraction of having to watch my footholds and allows me to proceed at my preferred speed.

Sight. I read somewhere a quarter of the total computing power of the brain is used up by the optical system. Not that remarkable when one considers it produces concise three-dimensional, moving, colour pictures. But I've found the receipt of constantly and rapidly, shifting images can, even in a short period, quite exhaust me. I assume it must be the continuous, fast data inflow changes which demand a matching response from my brain.

Examples: certain television programmes employ close-up filming techniques, rapidly switching from scene to scene. Some of these I've found so distressing I've been unable to watch for more than a few seconds. Again, being in a moving crowd for half an hour has the same tiring effect.

For many years I've been fully aware of this effect and of course, it's often possible to shut my eyes and walk away. But it's another reason why I avoid the cinema, or similar; there's no point in paying for my own discomfort.

Sound.   Another   source   of   information bombardment, — at times quite literally it seems — is sound. During waking hours it's becoming more and more difficult to find 'peace and quiet' for any sustained period around built-up areas. The huge increase in all forms of mechanised transport and machinery has ramped up the volume of background noise and made it continuous in some places.

Allied to this, more and more people seem unable to exist without continuous television or radio output, often with excessive volume. And it's irritating that much   noise   is   created   unthinkingly   with   no consideration of its effect on others.

Unlike excessive visual input, it's not easy, if not impossible, to switch off the noise barrage when outside the home. This can become most distressing during a major manic episode when the problem is amplified by the 'enhanced hearing' effect.

Sleep. I attach great importance to the quantity and quality of sleep and its function as an indicator of the approach of a manic episode.

It's accepted that sleep needs vary widely from person to person and may decrease with age. Whatever the average, currently I need six to seven hours relaxed sleep to be in a fit condition for the next day. I therefore take every practical action to achieve this ideal: silence, dark room, right temperature, comfortable bed, amount of covering, and a regular 24-hour cycle.

If I fail to get my normal sleep I'll be tired, irritable and humourless the next day. And, after a really bad night, my ability to concentrate is substantially reduced, the temples of my head feel bruised, and I really have to struggle to get through the daylight hours.

In my early years, my mother's obsession with sleep clearly affected my thinking, but I no longer worry just because I've had a bad night. But that doesn't alter the fact that I'm still unable to function properly, and can feel quite unwell if deprived of most of my sleep for any reason.

I'm fully aware the above comments could apply to anyone, but I get the impression my deterioration from sleep deprivation is more acute and prolonged than 'normal' people.

A punch. Any intense, short-lived, stress input not only raises my head temperature sharply, but can feel like a physical punch to the head. Typical work examples are: an urgent request to sort out a problem immediately, or request to construct a complex design to a short deadline. Arguments, driving mishaps, or near accidents, and similar highly charged incidents have the same effect.

The best example, and by far my most memorable incident of this type, took place at work some years ago. My office had two doors, one for regular use and the other clearly marked 'No Entrance', but kept usable as a fire escape. All staff were aware of, and respected, this situation.

After a period I relaxed my mental guard over the second door, trusting I'd not be interrupted from that source. Then one day a stranger in the building got lost and, frustrated, barged through the second door.

The shock to my system was so great it reached actual pain. I stood up, shaking, clamping my hands to my temples for relief, as my head temperature soared. Effectively, it seemed the shock had pierced my brain's defences, like a knife inflicted physical injury. (Fortunately, as far as the intruder was concerned, I was also rendered speechless and unable to voice my feelings!)

As these sudden stress inputs arrive without warning, there's nothing I can do to defend myself. But when it does happen I've trained myself to relax mind and body completely and try to let the distress play itself out.

Periods of concentration. Thankfully, I'm never likely to take aptitude tests again, but that embarrassing experience has made me extremely cautious when faced with any similar situation. Concentration, and its effect on tiring my brain, are areas I now keep to the forefront of my mind. As well as the intense focusing of the mind on one subject, this can also mean being 'confined' for a lengthy period on the same area of mental activity, such as driving a car.

In principle, I try and avoid any situation where I'm obliged to concentrate continuously, or intensely, for what I think might be an excessive period. At work, there's often no way I can avoid these pressures but now (nearing retirement!) I simply refuse to try and meet unreasonable deadlines.

When I'm working on a big project I try to chop it up into small pieces and treat each bit as a separate exercise: selecting a component, entering data on the word processor, speaking to a supplier. Then, every hour or so, I walk away from my desk, stroll round the factory, get a drink, perhaps go outside; just to divert my mind briefly from the subject.

If I go to a meeting with clients I can't of course dictate its speed or length. But often, with younger people present, things tend to zip along and this can cause me problems. When I start feeling really uncomfortable, my only escape is to say I don't feel well and go outside for a few minutes.

Socially, I steer clear of activities I believe, or know, involves intense mental effort, such as playing chess, card games like bridge, quizzes and the like. Anything in fact, which leads to me trying to speed up my thought processes and/or fast search my memory.

Protecting the memory. I've long thought that holding too much detail in the memory can be a source of stress. So I write notes when I can, then try to forget the subject to clear out my memory. And as already mentioned at work I, 'bin the junk' reserving use of my memory only for significant professional knowledge and experience.

This concept, though developed for work, I also employ at home. As well as keeping lists of things to be done, I also keep receipts, invoices and all paperwork associated with items bought and jobs done. By keeping a record, this allows me to relax and clear unwanted details out of my mind.

Burning off adrenaline. I suspect it's true that when tensed up, you can burn off surplus adrenaline by undertaking some suitably stressful activity. True or false, I'm sure that for me to attempt this and get the balance right, is well beyond my abilities. And of course, failure would certainly lead to an increase in my tension level.

In my case, the attempt would be less likely to succeed because I might be in or near a manic episode. At these times my judgement is distorted, likely to further muddy the waters. So I've always stuck to my basic defence against mania, staying cool and ducking and diving to avoid stress and excess tension.

I can only recall one occasion when, unintentionally, I burnt off the adrenaline in spectacularly successful way.

In the late '80s I was called in to play a League cricket match when near retirement from the game. At the start I felt awful; very hot-headed, dispirited and unable to concentrate. Wishing to do no more than sit and rest, when my team batted first I asked to be put at the bottom of the order.

As luck would have it, we lost wickets quickly and after an hour I had to go into bat in a dire situation. The bowlers were two youngsters flinging the ball down quite sharply and as I took guard I knew I'd have to quickly stoke up my reactions to avoid injury, let alone stay at the crease. I managed to do this for about forty minutes and made a useful contribution to the club's score.

In mental terms what I'd had to do, every half minute or so, was to concentrate intensely and then react physically as fast as I was could for a fraction of a second. All this of course, was driven by a real fear of injury.

When I was out and got back to the pavilion I felt like a new man. My head was cool and clear and I felt relaxed and in top form. It had been a unique and remarkable experience.

Rapid chat. While first working on this text it occurred to me there was an aspect of my behaviour I hadn't considered before; the technique of rapid fire chat used since my twenties.

For over thirty years I've used this style of speech on a regular basis and I'm now sure it must have contributed to my stress level, if only for the fact it must've been speeding up my brain. Since this danger dawned on me I've tried to maintain a moderate, measured delivery at all times.

An obvious advantage of this is that now, in the run-up to a manic episode, I can become aware of a speed-up of my speech. This is a useful indicator, particularly if I start to use colourful language with the odd swear word, at an inappropriate time.

(2) MANIC EPISODES

In this section I detail my understanding of the components of the manic episode and the way the cycle unfolds, for what has been the major on-going problem in my life since my first breakdown in '79.

When I first started going through manic episodes — I didn't even know what they were called — I can best describe it metaphorically as being propelled at breakneck speed through a dark, convoluted tunnel, then to suddenly wander out for a stroll in a sunlit meadow. I had no idea what was going on or what to expect and on the many occasions I went into the delusive state, this caused added fear and bewilderment.

It seems the various elements in the build-up phase of a manic episode all combine together and occur more or less simultaneously. Initially it was impossible to separate the different effects, but with the experience of many cycles I began to recognise the individual components, like unravelling a ball of string.

That's an understatement; in fact I developed an iron determination to get to grips with the problem by analysing every aspect of the process. The driving force behind this was the naked fear of 'losing my marbles', or 'going over the top', regularly or even permanently. To me it was a desperate imperative to find out what was going on and what I could do to keep my mind intact.

A manic episode is distressing, even painful at times, and certainly exhausting. The intensity of a sub-delusive episode can go from being a short period of 'speeding up' with broken sleep, to several weeks with all the symptoms I describe below. I've always been prepared to live with these if necessary, provided I avoided the delusive state and remained 'in control' of my mind.

I've read of the full-blown delusive episodes being called miniature nervous breakdowns and by their nature recalling them accurately is almost impossible. It's easy to exaggerate how many episodes in this category I've been through, but if I had to make a broad estimate I'd say between five and fifteen.

Over the years I've become steadily more aware of, or sensitive to, the behaviour and stresses I believe may bring on an episode. I regard my home as my base, where I have all the conditions available to stay on a stable keel, or 'cool down' if necessary. I'm sure I've developed neuroses and phobias over the years, but my automatic consideration now, about any event outside home, is not simply whether I'll enjoy it but whether I'll be able to handle whatever mental pressures may be involved.

I stumbled through the first episodes with no idea what was happening. Then gradually over the years I began to recognise repeated, specific features in each episode and started to sort out and separate the individual components. I continued to refine my understanding till about the mid-90's, since when I've had no reason to change or add to my analysis. Without undue arrogance I now believe I've learnt all there is to know about the process.

From the early days, I became aware that an episode is, time-wise, a clearly defined cycle: accelerating into the tunnel, then flopping out into the meadow, to return to normality. Of course the length of each cycle varies greatly; a very mild one might last three days, an average one around ten days, and a serious 'deeply embedded' one can take several months.

The real problem in trying to handle a manic episode, even now, is that I never realise it's happening till after it's started. And then whatever I might try to do, I can't stop the process unfolding. The only forewarning I sometimes get is the loss of my regular sleeping pattern.

I should add there's always been the option of using tranquillisers, though in practice, I've had to rule them out because of their effect on my driving. That aside, I've managed to avoid using them not just because of my antipathy to addictive drugs, but when I tried them for a period I disliked the warm muzzy feeling they induced. This I felt, contaminated the 'quality time' between episodes and blurred my judgement of my state of mind at any time.

For several years I took tranquillisers as soon as I became aware I was starting an episode, but invariably it was too late to have any effect till after the peak. And it's the pre-peak or tunnel period that's by far the more distressing.

In this part of the account, I detail my understanding of the various components of a manic episode, from starting to 'go high', through the tunnel and back to normality. I've no idea whether my experiences match those of others, but from a few snatches of written description and the odd anecdote from friends, it's possible they do.

Though my ability to think calmly during an episode is lost, there's usually been one or two incidents, or moments, which made me pause for thought and realise that odd things were happening. Over repeated episodes and in haphazard fashion, I've managed to separate and identify the individual components in spite of the racing confusion.

When I go into a manic episode everything speeds up though I usually don't notice this initially. As I move into the tunnel most of the components I list below seem to start functioning, giving the impression they're all happening together.

When I'm near the peak of a major episode I tend to focus intensely on one subject, losing track of the outside world and my normal daily habits. This continuous, narrow concentration can become slightly depressive and when the peak is passed it's a relief to be able to switch my mind freely to other things.

I've already said that the manic episodes I went through before taking lithium, were generally much worse than since. But to help me unravel the process, being thrown in at the deep end with the worst cycles had one advantage; it provided me with multiple, clearly defined, experiences often into serious delusions, from which to start climbing the learning curve.

The knowledge I've acquired doesn't alter the course of events, but it makes it easier for me if I know what's going on and roughly where I am in the cycle. It also allows me to warn others and ask for an element of understanding for my 'eccentric' behaviour.

And importantly, my original fear of an episode has now largely evaporated. I'm confident I know the process and what's likely to happen next. At the same time I know the cycle will be exhausting, even more so as I get older. I can only hope that relief, the sunny meadow, is not too far ahead.

The specific components of the manic episodes I've experienced are, in any order:

Speeding up. Clearly, this is the major component of the manic episode, the one aspect of mania about which most people have some concept. Its effect is the most powerful and obvious signal of the start of an episode, yet impossible to counteract short of heavy drugs or an immediate rest cure, perhaps. Once started, it seems my mind races along out of control as if drawn by some outside force.

Though I'll get exhausted, I'll be unable to slow down mentally or, in any sense, 'take a break'. When I'm not physically doing anything I'm still likely to be thinking hard about a particular subject, tending to become more obsessive and focused. (Even my daily body clock speeds up; I find myself doing routine things an hour or two earlier).

At work I panic about getting everything done, as if there were no tomorrow, incapable of planning ahead and with no time for the broader picture. Confusingly, reality can become reversed; my colleagues appearing to be rushing around the place, so much so that at times I've asked them to, 'slow down!'

When I've become aware of what's happening, I'm powerless to take any corrective action and simply get swept along towards the peak. In recent years, when I've twigged what's going on, I've tried to ease the stress by 'letting go', pushing work away or setting back any deadline. This releases the pressure somewhat but I still have to complete the cycle.

Generally, as I get nearer the peak, my racing mind tends to focus exclusively on one subject, pushing all others into the background. The deeper the episode the more intense this is. The subject may be something quite mundane, a humorous incident perhaps, or something more complex and serious involving intense thought and concentration.

To digress on this topic, it's easy to see how the intensity, continuity and power of thought, frantic or otherwise, by someone in the manic phase must occasionally produce something brilliant. In the famous example of Isaac Newton, no doubt the sheer power and unremitting concentration of his thinking helped produce his works of creative genius. And the scale and complexity of his ideas probably meant he went through many episodes before he satisfied himself that he'd arrived at the right conclusions.

At the same time, the massive efforts totally exhausted his mind, driving him into sleep deprivation, delusions and despair. But as his written works reveal, the intense concentration and obsessive attention to detail produced a near-perfect final text.

Moving from the sublime to the ridiculous, I've sometimes written-up a humorous story during a manic episode. In doing this I've found the driving continuous thought, focused on one simple subject, has not only been exhausting but is effectively a form of perfectionism. Always my article has been highly polished, the frequent prior changes just going round in circles. Reviewing my final text afterwards in a stable state, I usually conclude there's nothing much I could improve on.

The combination of speed, with concentration on one subject, tends to shut out reality as I hurtle through the tunnel longing for the end. In a sense the glimmer of, 'the light at the end of the tunnel', marks the peak of the episode and the beginning of relief. My mind flops out, exhausted by the mental effort which is exacerbated by the loss of quality sleep during this period.

I've also noticed that this part of an episode is the one time I can become depressed. I'm sure this is due to the exhaustion from the continuous effort, inability to relax and slow down, plus the realisation that once again, I'm going through a manic episode.

Appearance. My physical appearance and personality alter during episodes and Carol, with long experience, has helped me list these. I lose my sense of humour and sparkle, become quiet and introspective, sometimes despondent. I develop heavy, dark rings under the eyes and exhibit a watery, glazed expression. And I often sit or stand staring vacantly into space, lost in my own thoughts and oblivious of those around me.

Head temperature. I've always regarded my head temperature, described earlier, as the key indicator of stress. At its mildest the 'hot head' feeling can be just a feeling of slight warmth across the forehead; at worst it's like a hot clamp compressing the forehead and temple area. It's a continuous, reliable indicator and as I go into an episode invariably my temperature and tension rise.

The 'staring' effect. A theory I have — almost certainly crackpot! — is that a surfeit of adrenaline (or whatever the chemicals are) created during a manic episode, distorts the optical system of the brain. Certainly what does happen is that my perception of people is altered such that they appear to be staring at me. I'm sure this is nothing to do with personality change, simply a temporary, chemically induced effect.

Initially others appear slightly glassy-eyed; as the episode intensifies I think they're gazing at me in wide-eyed amazement, readily construed as adoration. This effect I've found most disconcerting and embarrassing, in the early days leading to me believing I was someone rather special. (The term 'delusions of grandeur', long associated with mania, must surely be connected with this phenomenon.)

To add to the confusion, with usual discretion relaxed, I would sometimes exacerbate the situation by making some outrageous 'off the wall' comment. This would trigger a genuinely astounded reaction from the listener.

It took some years before I understood and got to grips with this effect. Obviously, all I have to do is ignore it but, as I've said before, it's never easy to fathom this out and think logically in the confusion of an episode.

Enhanced hearing. What I call 'enhanced hearing' is perhaps the most pernicious effect during the manic episode cycle. It causes considerable discomfort in itself and of course, it's rarely possible to 'turn off' incoming noise. And it appears, few people have much idea of the distress excessive noise can cause others.

In the normal 'hardened' state it seems as if there's a shield protecting the nervous system, which cushions the shock of a sudden noise. It also provides a layer of insulation to reduce the intensity of incoming sounds to a level more acceptable to the brain.

During an episode (and similar to the 'staring effect'), 'enhanced hearing' appears to be a chemically-induced alteration to hearing. It seems the normal shield has been stripped away and I become hypersensitive to incoming sound, which is somehow amplified in my unprotected brain.

In this state, a door being slammed can not only make me jump, but actually cause physical pain. In another situation, the enhanced noise effect has overwhelmed me and I've resorted to clamping hands over ears, when others around are unconcerned.

The effect doesn't lead to any noticeably strange behaviour and therefore no reaction from people around. But with few even aware of the problem, one can't expect much understanding or assistance. A classic example of this problem was with my own family; for years I was told, 'don't be so silly', when I complained the television was too loud.

To further emphasise this point I recall two significant incidents, when I'm sure enhanced hearing played a crucial, destructive part.

When first in hospital during the 'Durham event', I couldn't sleep at all because of the noise in the ward.

This was regarded as quite normal by the staff, who had no idea of the effect it was having on me. Had they done so and moved me to a quieter place, it's possible I'd have snatched enough sleep to prevent my decline into delusions.

Then, I refer to the situation at the height of my second breakdown detailed earlier, when I was 'boiling hot' and desperate for sleep. If I'd been able to snatch an hour or two, undisturbed by the billiard balls, there's an outside chance — with sedatives — the crisis could have been defused.

Walking. I've written elsewhere about the valuable therapeutic aspects of walking, for cooling my head down as well as exercise. But during a manic episode it's also a useful physical indicator of my state of mind.

As I approach the peak I walk faster than normal, mind focused elsewhere, often unaware of where I'm going. In this mood I'm likely to walk too far, mind racing ahead of body. Ridiculous though it may seem, on one occasion I got quite lost and on another, I was walking so fast I pulled a leg muscle!

After the peak I find myself walking slower, lacking in energy, and likely to cover less than my usual ground. (After a really intense delusive cycle I've found myself struggling to go much more than a hundred yards.)

For these reasons I've found it an advantage to have a regular route, to allow me to measure my performance against the norm. Only when I'm 'balanced' between manic episodes, do I walk in a relaxed way, a comfortable, manageable distance, needing no conscious adjustment of pace or route.

Speech and Shock. This is a symptom of the manic condition that can be readily perceived by others. My voice rises slightly in pitch, I speak faster and become more talkative. My tongue is loosened, sometimes slipping into colourful language and indiscretions. The famous example is Groucho Marx, with his rapid-fire wit, joke-telling and instant responses.

All this is a consequence of my brain speeding up. I tend to 'pounce' on someone's words and spew back a lightning fast, ill-considered, response. Often I've seen surprise register on the person's face by the speed of it all.

In addition, after an animated conversation which has raised my head temperature, I tremble on the brink of breaking with emotion, whatever the subject matter. And if the effort excites my brain too much I can go into a narcoleptic faint, my body goes limp and everything cuts out for a split second. Usually, my brain automatically takes that as a warning signal, so I stop talking and rest to allow myself time to 'harden up'.

During the worst episodes I've sometimes gone into a full 'drop dead' faint, when my whole nervous system has tripped out. Usually, as soon as I've hit the floor the impact has brought me round but of course, it does alarm others.

An amusing anecdote on this was the time I went for a walk when very 'high', close to delusion. Carol, worried about my condition, asked an old friend to go with me. As we passed a pub, he suggested we nip in for a swift half.

When we opened the door I was hit by the heat and noise of the packed bar, which triggered a faint and I collapsed, sprawling forward into the room. I came round quickly and scrambled to my feet, but the landlord having seen the incident, was adamant:

'He's not to be served; I'm not having drunks in my pub!

Sleeping. My mother was obsessive about sleep; a 'good night's sleep' or an 'early night', was her answer to every illness including it would seem, a broken leg. By the time I'd managed to adjust my childhood indoctrination to a more balanced view, I'd arrived at broken nights caused by mania.

I rely heavily now on my sleeping pattern as the clearest indicator of my state of mind. Also, of vital importance, it can be the one advance warning of the approach of a manic episode.

I try to maintain a regular, daily cycle — without sleeping pills — in optimum conditions, at all times. When my sleep is fully relaxed and mostly unbroken I can virtually guarantee that I'm in the balanced state between episodes.

From the start of a manic episode my sleeping rhythm is broken, usually by waking several times, the first earlier than normal. Progressively, as the episode develops I wake earlier and earlier, till I may get less than an hour's sleep after going to bed.

This short initial sleep is I understand, just recovering from physical tiredness and not the essential, deep nourishing sleep one needs. Whatever the reason, when this starts to happen I know I'm over-stressed.

When I've woken, or can't get to sleep, if I lie too long in bed I develop a mild headache. So I always get out of bed, go somewhere else, and sit in an upright position. I may have a drink, perhaps read and usually after half an hour or so, I start to feel drowsy. Then I go to bed and try again.

If this fails and I stay awake I'll repeat the process and, unless I'm really 'high', usually snatch an hour or two before dawn. Nowadays, when I get the occasional bad night I try not to worry about it, reckoning to catch up the next night.

Thankfully, for the last ten years at least, I've avoided reaching such a tensed state that I've had to resort to sleeping pills. But I accept now that if that did happen, there's no alternative to some sort of medication to relax my mind and allow it to get essential deep sleep. Otherwise, it's the downhill spiral into total exhaustion, delusions, and all that follows.

Neatness. Working in an office, over the years I've developed my own paperwork systems, procedures and so on. I always keep lists of work to be done and write notes quickly in block capitals, a clear way of communicating.

One of the first visible signs of the 'Speeding up' effect and onset of an episode, is that these lists become untidy. My writing becomes scrawly and eventually, illegible, with sentences tailing off unfinished.

Because my mind is starting to race I don't always notice this deterioration initially, but when I've had occasion to re-read something just written, the penny usually drops. Being a visual indicator it's that much more effective and over the years it's been a regular means of registering I'm in an episode and given a clue to its intensity.

Delusions   With a slow but steady build-up of confidence since my second breakdown,
plus experience gained, I can't believe I'll allow myself to get near the delusive state in future.   That said, of course there's always some combination of circumstances that may await me, sufficient to penetrate all my defences.

In recent years my episodes have been hypomanic rather than manic; though I might dwell over-long on one subject for a period near the peak, it could be called perfectionism rather than obsession.   I don't believe I've gone 'over the top' into the true delusive state since I started lithium in '87, but memories of those earlier days still provide a compelling incentive to avoid any recurrence.

I've already outlined the process: mental exhaustion, fuelled by unbroken, high speed thought, continuous concentration and sleeplessness which, if intense enough, drives me 'over the top' into the delusive state.   And I'm painfully aware that once I go too far down that road I'm into a vicious spiral that's almost impossible to break out of, before total exhaustion.

In the early days, my instincts were to try and cover up what was really happening, so that people around me would be unaware of the problem.   This of course, was precisely the wrong thing to do and prevented me getting help when needed.

I'm now persuaded that, in spite of my antipathy to drugs, when spiralling towards the delusive state the best option is to take a powerful sedative. Apart perhaps from a full rest cure, nothing else will allow me to break out of the downward spiral. Without that, the natural route is so protracted, distressing and exhausting, plus all the problems generated by delusions, there's a fair chance it could lead to another visit to a mental hospital.

I'm able to write now, with the hint of a smile, of three incidents relating to delusions during powerful manic episodes from the early '80s.

During one episode I became obsessed with neatness and precision. I would walk about the house continually looking for any picture, ornament or pot plant not exactly centred on the shelf or sill. I extended this to the office, generating some strange looks from colleagues who, thankfully, figured out there was something wrong.

On another occasion, when we had a small billiard table in the lounge, Carol got up one morning to find all the household toiletries, lavatory brushes and cleaning fluids, neatly arranged on it. I'd done this during the night and I've been unable to remember my reason for so doing.

Perhaps the most dramatic episode was when I collected all the cheque books, credit cards and bank statements in the house, went for a walk and threw them into someone else's dustbin. At the practical level, this presented Carol with an immediate problem as she had no means of buying the weekly shopping!

This last delusion appears to have an obvious sub-conscious meaning, but I've never analysed or worried about any of them since. More importantly perhaps, I've never re-visited the same subject again, so I don't think I have any neurotic tendencies.

The peak.   I can't think of any technical way to describe the peak of a manic episode and can only resort to a metaphor similar to one I used earlier. It's like the mind switching from being an arrow hurtling uncontrolled through a dark tunnel, to suddenly become a plateful of warm, soggy spaghetti in a bright, sunlit room.

I've no idea when to expect the peak when in the tunnel, apart from the vague feeling I might soon be seeing the light. And I'm never aware precisely when the peak takes place, or has taken place, other than the distinct switch-over of mood. If it's not at a specific time it must be a short period or when I'm asleep. Emotionally, after a delusive manic episode, the release from tension accompanied by total mental exhaustion can be quite orgasmic, no other word is apposite.

Coming down from the peak.   After the peak, apart from exhaustion, the recovery phase is straight forward.   The key feeling is a wondrous sense of calm, slowness and absence of any pressure as time floats pleasantly by.   This totally relaxed sensation spreads to the body, like the after-glow from a thorough massage.

At the same time I'm emotionally weak and drained, with tears ready to flow at any hint of sentiment. Also, I'll be ultra sensitive to any perceived minor slight or discourtesy, unable to dismiss it from my mind.

My eyesight returns to normality; I can see people clearly again and read their expressions properly, rather than through a distorting fog of tension and adrenaline.

Another effect is that my mind feels as if it's swimming in surplus adrenaline. Like a highly flammable fluid, even a mildly taxing event can rapidly drive my head temperature up. For example, a ten minute enjoyable, mildly animated conversation, can cause my forehead to become baking hot, to the point of sweating. Yet a following similar period of rest and quiet will pull the temperature right down again.

Given the right balance of rest and activity, my mind steadily toughens up till I reach normal 'hardness' and am ready to face outside pressures again. Like a physical injury, I suspect the best technique to accelerate recovery would be to steadily exercise the mind for progressively longer periods. But I've always reckoned it would be impossible to judge that correctly without specialist supervision, so I simply let nature take its course.

After the worst manic episodes my mind would be utterly exhausted, literally quite unable to add two and two together, or remember the answer. My mental processes would seem to be mired in treacle and I'd be unable to concentrate on anything for more than a few seconds. Only those who've actually experienced this level of mental exhaustion can possibly appreciate what it's like.

Some examples: I couldn't remember how to tie my shoelaces up; it was pointless reading because I couldn't remember the previous sentence; doing a simple chore, I'd stop after a short time as I'd forgotten what I was supposed to be doing.

There's many more examples like that but to hasten recovery it's clearly necessary to push things along to some extent. The best judge of how far and fast to go is always my head temperature. Walking is also a valuable guide in this phase: the speed and distance I cover indicating the strength, or otherwise, of my recovery.

My sleeping pattern remains broken for a week or more; but length of the first sleep usually increases each night. After a bad manic episode, this sleep would be deep, unbroken, blissful even, leaving me wonderfully refreshed the next day.

I believe that, in theory, at the end of the recovery period I return to a mentally balanced, normal condition. (Without being too bleakly pessimistic, I also assume it's the point from which I start the run-up to the next manic episode!)

(3) The social problem

What I call 'the social problem' is in a way the most exasperating aspect of mania. It's the fact that no-one I've met outside the medical world has any understanding of the subject and probably won't even have heard of it.

Thankfully, my family and close friends have achieved a fair understanding of its practical effects by now and know how to 'handle me' during a manic phase. But trying to explain to others in a social context, even the gist of what it's about has always been beyond me.

My frustration is partly explained by the rarity of the condition; about one percent of the population suffer from some form of manic depression, of which less than one in ten are manic only. Certainly I've never met or heard about, anyone with precisely the same problem as me, even when in mental hospital.

Mania being essentially unheard of leads to a lack of any real understanding, so my attempts over the years to find a shorthand method of giving its 'bullet points' have met with little success. People have an outline knowledge of the common physical ailments and many disabilities or injuries are visible. But when I walk into a room full of strangers, there's simply no way I can easily explain the basics of my mental problem or state of mind, should it be necessary.

Typical social events I like to arrange with friends: joining them at golf, an evening meal, meeting in a pub, a day at a cricket match, are all occasions for enjoyment. No one is going to thank me, or be that interested, if I take them aside to give a lesson in the basics of mania. And even close friends can't quite understand, if I opt out of a much sought-after entertainment, solely because of mania.

It doesn't help that the language and words related to mania can be confusing. If broaching the subject, I've learnt from much experience never to mention 'depression' or its derivatives. When I have done so, the listener beams a knowing smile of recognition, before listing a catalogue of people and events they've known suffering from various forms of depression. There's much potential sympathy of course, but minds tend to be closed to mania as a fundamentally different problem.

'Manic', maniac', and 'manic behaviour are all in common use, and portray someone rushing around or behaving violently in the physical sense. This basic picture suggests two components of a manic episode, 'speeding up' and 'rapid speech', but doesn't touch on the many less obvious aspects.

Some years ago I tried to 'dumb down' my description using only words such as 'tension' or 'stress', but that only generates mild sympathy and stock *clichés* such as, 'tell me about it', or, 'you and me both'.

Nowadays, I no longer attempt to discuss the principles of mania to anyone in a social context. Apart from the communication problem, people rarely consider that we all have different mental strengths and stamina, in the same way that some people can run a mile in four minutes, others take ten. Hopefully my conversational skills suggest a degree of intelligence, but my brain's stamina and ability to cope with stress is another matter.

My reason for wanting to explain mania to others is so I can offer a true explanation for turning down invitations, or avoiding certain things. I don't like lying, ——a stress in itself — or to appear unfriendly or anti-social. And simply to say I don't like excessive heat, noise, and so on, sounds pretty lame when few enjoy those conditions anyway.

Starting my adult life again, with the same problem, logically I'd opt for more leisurely pursuits: bird watching, hill climbing, train-spotting, or the like. These things don't involve intense mental activity and I could easily stay calm without having to think about it. But I can't change course now without abandoning most of my life-long friends and interests, something I'm loathe to contemplate.

The basic mania problem is compounded further in that the conditions I need to protect myself, are contrary to the social thrust of the day. I get the impression the world is speeding up, with more travelling and physical activity undertaken, while attention spans shorten. Also, images projected by the media also tend to move in one direction: fast, intense, instant, exciting and pressurised.

In sport, commentators praise competitors who are aggressive and focused and it's considered impossible to perform effectively at the highest level unless, 'the adrenaline's up'. Apparently, people are looking for a bigger 'buzz': bungee jumping, scuba diving, paint ball, stock car racing, para-gliding, inter-active computer games and so on. This trend I suggest, is quite contrary to the needs of the mania sufferer.

With so many old cricket and other pals, some of over forty years standing, I still much enjoy the odd get-together. And my love of anecdotes, stories and repartee means I can still contribute to the fun as in the past. However, the lack of understanding of mania, coupled with the social trends, mean I'm not just opting, but being forced to abandon this activity to adopt a quieter, less stimulating life.

So far I've tackled this conundrum by good old British compromise: I trade off the enjoyment of a lively social event involving, 'putting my head in the fire', with the price to be paid in terms of head temperature, over-tension, lost sleep and feeling simply awful the next day.

Obviously, as time passes I shall increasingly favour the relatively boring, calm, existence; I must face the fact that with the ageing process, the threshold of discomfort and distress will be continually reducing.

(4) Definitions of mania

During the time I've written this account I've looked for definitions of mania, on the internet or elsewhere, as a matter of interest. Apparently there are two main international standards used to classify the disorder: ICD10 is generally used in the UK and Europe. DSM IV is produced by the American Psychiatric Association and I understand is probably the most comprehensive definitions available anywhere.
I thought it would be useful to compare my experiences with these formal definitions so for this purpose I've used the DSM IV standard.

The DSM IV definitions are shown in *italics* with my comment or reaction to each item thereafter.

3.3   What is mania?

Criteria for Manic Episode (DSM – 1V, p.332)
A. *A distinct period of abnormally and persistently elevated, expansive, or irritable mood, lasting at least 1 week (or any duration if hospitalisation is necessary).*

Basically I agree; in my case elevated mood probably more apparent to an observer than to me. Irritability almost always due to tiredness. The duration of at least one week certainly applies to the major manic episodes. A relatively minor cycle could be completed in only three days.

B. *During the period of mood disturbance, three (or more) of the following symptoms have persisted (four if the mood is only irritable) and have been present to a significant degree:*

(1) inflated self-esteem or grandiosity
1   No, never. Again, these may appear to be the case, relative to my normal behaviour, to an observer.
(2) decreased need for sleep (e.g., feels rested after only 3 hours of sleep)
I may appear to need less sleep only because I can't relax enough to get it naturally due to over-tension and exhaustion. Driven by the 'speeding up' effect, this may appear energetic to others and account for the comment, 'feels rested after only 3 hours of sleep'.

(3) more talkative than usual or pressure to keep talking

True; 'rapid speech' and the 'speeding up effect' are the most obvious symptoms. Fast and excessive speech can easily be discerned by others with 'instant' responses and a tendency to digress and go into far more detail than necessary.

(4) flight of ideas or subjective experience that thoughts are racing

Broadly true, though normally in an episode I have one idea which may or may not be fantastical.

(5) distractibility (i.e., attention too easily drawn to unimportant or irrelevant external stimuli)

Not really though it may appear to be the case. During the speeding up phase the mind is super-active, mostly concentrated on the goal(s) described in *(4)* and *(6)*. But if my mind 'takes a breather' from the main subject it's pursuing, it will look for something else to occupy it.

(6) increase in goal-directed activity (either socially, at work or school, or sexually) or psychomotor agitation

To the first part, my answer would be similar to *(4)* above. The drive to achieve something is all-consuming and exhausting, whether the goal is sensible or otherwise.

(Unable to understand the 'psychomotor agitation' part!)

(7) excessive involvement in pleasurable activities that have a high potential for painful consequences (e.g., engaging in unrestrained

buying sprees, sexual indiscretions, or foolish business investments)
No, never. My personality, apart from its pessimism, is essentially practical. Any thought of doing something I couldn't afford, unusual or indiscreet, would be over-ruled by my 'intellect'. Also and importantly, as soon as I've realised I'm in a manic episode, I've consciously avoided taking any important decisions for the obvious reason that my usual judgement could be distorted.

C. *The symptoms do not meet criteria for a Mixed Episode.*
Agree no. (in as far as I can understand the definition of a Mixed Episode)

D. *The mood disturbance is sufficiently severe to cause marked impairment in occupational functioning or in usual social activities or relationships with others, or to necessitate hospitalisation to prevent harm to self or others, or there are psychotic features.*
Without doubt, a bad manic episode does impair my ability to work normally. To that end I've always tried to explain the gist of the problem to colleagues to prepare them in advance. With their co-operation and understanding (which I've always received), I can avoid aspects of my job which could be adversely affected by my behaviour during an episode. In particular, I try to avoid speaking direct to clients, mainly because of my speech and what I might say could be commercially

indiscreet. At the social level, this is a problem I've already discussed in a previous section. (I've never needed to be hospitalised, as the Americans say, to prevent harm to myself or others.

E. *The symptoms are not due to the direct physiological effects of a substance (e.g., a drug of abuse, a medication, or other treatments) or a general medical condition (e.g., hyperthyroidism).*

I've never taken non-prescription drugs and the only long-term prescription ones I take now are lithium, carbamazapine and thyroxine as detailed earlier in this paper.
In the early '80s I took, up to the prescribed limit, various tranquillisers such as Largactil and Stelazine to try and counter the effects of a manic episode. Later I took Pimozide but I've not used this, or any similar drug, since '92.) I'm not aware of any other general medical condition.

The DSM manual then continues with the definitions of hypomania. I quote in italics with my comments following:

3.4 *What is hypomania?*

Hypomania means, literally, "mild mania."
It's sometimes difficult to draw a distinct line between "manic" and "hypomanic," as "marked impairment" is a necessarily subjective evaluation.

Also, one of the reasons that bipolar disorder often has a delayed diagnosis may be that hypomanic episodes are often overlooked amid the "Sturm und Drang" of adolescence and early adulthood.
The associated features of mania are present in Hypomanic Episodes, except that delusions are never present and all other symptoms are *generally* less severe than they would be in Manic Episodes.

Criteria for Hypomanic Episode (DSM-IV, p. 338)

A. A distinct period of persistently elevated, expansive, or irritable mood, lasting throughout at least 4 days, that is clearly different from the usual non-depressed mood.

B. During the period of mood disturbance, three (or more) of the following symptoms have persisted (four if the mood is only irritable) and have been present to a significant degree:
(1) inflated self-esteem or grandiosity
(2) decreased need for sleep (e.g., feels rested after only 3 hours of sleep)
(3) more talkative than usual or pressure to keep talking
(4) flight of ideas or subjective experience that thoughts are racing
(5) distractibility (i.e., attention too easily drawn to unimportant or irrelevant external stimuli)
(6) increase in goal-directed activity (either socially, at work or school, or sexually) or psychomotor agitation
(7) excessive involvement in pleasurable activities that have a high potential for painful consequences

(e.g., engaging in unrestrained buying sprees, sexual indiscretions, or foolish business investments)

C. The episode is associated with an unequivocal change in functioning that is uncharacteristic of the person when not symptomatic.

D. The disturbance in mood and the change in functioning are observable by others.

E. The episode is not severe enough to cause marked impairment in social or occupational functioning, or to necessitate hospitalisation, and there are no psychotic features.

F. The symptoms are not due to the direct physiological effects of a substance (e.g., a drug of abuse, a medication, or other treatment) or a general medical condition (e.g., hyperthyroidism).

These definitions seem to be for just a milder form of mania. I tend to simplify things by thinking that mania goes, or can go, into the delusive state ('over the top') whereas in hypomania the delusive state of mind is never reached. Since my second breakdown, when I started taking lithium, I believe I've never gone above the hypomanic state when going through manic episodes.

(5) Reflections

As I near retirement age the stresses and strains of earning my living have started to ease away, though I'm not exactly excited about my likely standard of living as a pensioner.

In the Introduction I mentioned the controversy in the psychiatric world about whether or not mania qualifies as a disease and obviously, I'm not knowledgeable enough on this to offer an expert opinion. But there's no doubt the frequency and intensity of my manic episodes have tailed off in recent years and this appears to run contemporaneously with the reduction in my job and financial pressures.

At the time of writing my last manic episode of any consequence was about three years ago and I've gained confidence that I can avoid any further in the foreseeable future. That doesn't of course exclude the possibility that I may be involved in some intensely stressful event or emergency, triggering a serious episode.

I'm now as sure as I can be that the mania I've had was initiated by my job and the environment in which I worked. My first breakdown then caused a permanent weakening of my brain, reducing my threshold for coping with stress or adverse mental conditions, to below the norm. So, for practical day-to-day handling of the problem, I've worked on the premise that my brain, in the physical sense anyway, is relatively over-sensitive and lacking in stamina.

Having survived, or muddled through, the early years of the initial delusive, manic episodes, I've built up an understanding of the stresses that initiate them and the process itself. This experience has enabled me to 'duck and dive' over the years to minimise the more distressing effects of mania. (I've been fortunate to have lived in a peaceful location and able to obtain quiet in my home when needed).

With the incidence and intensity of my manic episodes diminishing, particularly in recent years, in a slightly masochistic way, I'd be interested to know if, or how well, I could cope without lithium? I don't ever expect to be able to answer this; I've been strongly advised to continue taking lithium 'to the grave!'. There seems no point even considering ignoring this advice while as far as I know, my physical health has not been, and is not being, impaired in any noticeable way.

But in reflection, the repeated episodes have had a debilitating and negative psychological effect: I've become progressively less inclined to get into (what I think) might be stressful situations and more inclined to take the easy option. Though that doesn't really matter, my enjoyment of life has been somewhat reduced.

In recent years, with greater confidence of my understanding and ability to cope with mania, I've allowed myself to relax my guard in that area. At the same time, I've become acutely aware of the vital necessity of protecting my brain from over-tiredness. (Clearly also, I must assume my mental stamina will decline with age.)

It seems this exhaustion comes from some combination of normal tiredness, unbroken mental activity, excessive concentration, staying too long in an over-active environment, or continuous, intense inflow of sound and/or visual images.

Though this might appear to be a comparatively minor problem, when I've unwittingly over-stretched my brain, the resulting distress and pain have been worse than anything experienced during a manic episode, though over a shorter period. This revelation has surprised and shocked me.

My Diary notes for 2004 seem to indicate my basic troubles with mania may now be ending, though I think it's too early to say, with complete confidence, that I'm now 'a free man'. Clearly, my recent use of atenolol has had a major effect in eliminating the 'hot head' feeling and that, in itself, is an immense relief.

Finally, constructing this paper has been the most difficult writing exercise I've undertaken. Trying to commit something serious to paper has been a terrific challenge for an amateur scribbler. Whether the content is of any interest to anyone, I've no idea.

THE END